T0227018

Faces of Right Ventricular Failure

Guest Editors

JAMES A. GOLDSTEIN, MD
JONATHAN D. RICH, MD

CARDIOLOGY CLINICS

www.cardiology.theclinics.com

Consulting Editor
MICHAEL H. CRAWFORD, MD

May 2012 • Volume 30 • Number 2

SAUNDERS an imprint of ELSEVIER, Inc.

W.B. SAUNDERS COMPANY
A Division of Elsevier Inc.

1600 John F. Kennedy Blvd. • Suite 1800 • Philadelphia, PA 19103-2899

http://www.theclinics.com

CARDIOLOGY CLINICS Volume 30, Number 2
May 2012 ISSN 0733-8651, ISBN-13: 978-1-4557-3838-0

Editor: Barbara Cohen-Kligerman
Developmental Editor: Teia Stone

Cardiology Clinics (ISSN 0733-8651) is published quarterly by Elsevier Inc., 360 Park Avenue South, New York, NY 10010-1710. Months of issue are February, May, August, and November. Business and Editorial Offices: 1600 John F. Kennedy Blvd., Ste. 1800, Philadelphia, PA 19103-2899. Customer Service Office: 3251 Riverport Lane, Maryland Heights, MO 63043. Periodicals postage paid at New York, NY and additional mailing offices. Subscription prices are $305.00 per year for US individuals, $488.00 per year for US institutions, $150.00 per year for US students and residents, $373.00 per year for Canadian individuals, $606.00 per year for Canadian institutions, $432.00 per year for international individuals, $606.00 per year for international institutions and $212.00 per year for Canadian and international students/residents. To receive student/resident rate, orders must be accompanied by name of affiliated institution, data of term, and the *signature* of program/residency coordinator on institution letterhead. Orders will be billed at individual rate until proof of status is received. Foreign air speed delivery is included in all *Clinics* subscription prices. All prices are subject to change without notice. **POSTMASTER:** Send address changes to *Cardiology Clinics*, Elsevier Health Sciences Division, Subscription Customer Service, 3251 Riverport Lane, Maryland Heights, MO 63043. **Customer Service: 1-800-654-2452 (U.S. and Canada); 314-447-8871 (outside U.S. and Canada). Fax: 314-447-8029. E-mail: journalscustomerservice-usa@elsevier.com (for print support); journalsonlinesupport-usa@elsevier.com (for online support).**

Reprints. For copies of 100 or more, of articles in this publication, please contact the Commercial Reprints Department, Elsevier Inc., 360 Park Avenue South, New York, NY 10010-1710. Tel.: 212-633-3812; Fax: 212-462-1935; E-mail: reprints@elsevier.com.

Cardiology Clinics is also published in Spanish by McGraw-Hill Interamericana Editores S. A., P.O. Box 5-237, 06500, Mexico D. F., Mexico; in Portuguese by Reichmann and Alfonso Editores Rio de Janeiro, Brazil; and in Greek by Dimitrios P. Lagos, 8 Pondon Street, GR115-28 Ilissia, Greece.

Cardiology Clinics is covered in *MEDLINE/PubMed (Index Medicus), Excerpta Medica, The Cumulative Index to Nursing and Allied Health Literature* (CINAHL).

Printed and bound by CPI Group (UK) Ltd, Croydon, CR0 4YY

Transferred to Digital Print 2012

Contributors

CONSULTING EDITOR

MICHAEL H. CRAWFORD, MD
Professor of Medicine, University of California, San Francisco; Lucie Stern Chair in Cardiology and Chief of Clinical Cardiology, University of California, San Francisco Medical Center, San Francisco, California

GUEST EDITORS

JAMES A. GOLDSTEIN, MD
Director of Research and Education, Department of Cardiovascular Medicine, Beaumont Health System, Royal Oak, Michigan

JONATHAN D. RICH, MD
Assistant Professor of Medicine, Section of Cardiology, Department of Medicine, University of Chicago Medical Center, Chicago, Illinois

AUTHORS

CHRISTIAN CASTILLO, MD
Fellow, Division of Pulmonary and Critical Care Medicine, Duke University Medical Center, Durham, North Carolina

JENNIFER CONROY, MD, MBE
Cardiology Fellow, Zena and Michael A. Wiener Cardiovascular Institute and Marie-Josee and Henry R. Kravis Center for Cardiovascular Health, Mount Sinai Hospital, New York, New York

LOUIS J. DELL'ITALIA, MD
Division of Cardiovascular Disease, Birmingham Veterans Affairs Medical Center, Birmingham, Alabama

JAMES A. GOLDSTEIN, MD
Director of Research and Education, Department of Cardiovascular Medicine, Beaumont Health System, Royal Oak, Michigan

PAUL M. HASSOUN, MD
Professor of Medicine, Division of Pulmonary and Critical Care Medicine, Johns Hopkins University; Director, Pulmonary Hypertension Program, Johns Hopkins University, Baltimore, Maryland

WILLIAM E. HOPKINS, MD, FACC, FACP
Associate Professor, Department of Medicine, Cardiology Unit, University of Vermont College of Medicine; Pulmonary Hypertension and Adult Congenital Heart Disease Programs, Fletcher Allen Health Care, Burlington, Vermont

MORTON J. KERN, MD
Department of Cardiology, Long Beach Veterans Affairs Hospital, Long Beach, California

TODD M. KOLB, MD, PhD
Post-Doctoral Fellow, Division of Pulmonary and Critical Care Medicine, Johns Hopkins University, Baltimore, Maryland

JAGAT NARULA, MD, PhD
Director, Cardiovascular Imaging Program; Professor of Medicine/Cardiology, Zena and Michael A. Wiener Cardiovascular Institute and Marie-Josee and Henry R. Kravis Center for Cardiovascular Health, Mount Sinai School of Medicine; Mount Sinai Hospital, New York, New York

JONATHAN D. RICH, MD
Assistant Professor of Medicine, Section
of Cardiology, Department of Medicine,
University of Chicago Medical Center,
Chicago, Illinois

STUART RICH, MD
Section of Cardiology, Department of
Medicine, University of Chicago, Chicago,
Illinois

JAVIER SANZ, MD
Director of Cardiac MR/CT, Assistant
Professor of Medicine/Cardiology,
Zena and Michael A. Wiener
Cardiovascular Institute and Marie-Josee and
Henry R. Kravis Center for Cardiovascular
Health, Mount Sinai School of Medicine,
New York, New York

GABRIEL T. SAYER, MD
Cardiology Division, Department of Medicine,
Massachusetts General Hospital and Harvard
Medical School, Boston, Massachusetts

MARC J. SEMIGRAN, MD
Cardiology Division, Department of Medicine,
Massachusetts General Hospital and Harvard
Medical School, Boston, Massachusetts

VICTOR F. TAPSON, MD
Professor, Division of Pulmonary and
Critical Care Medicine; Director, Division of
Pulmonary, Allergy and Critical Care Medicine,
Pulmonary Vascular Disease Center,
Duke University Medical Center, Durham,
North Carolina

GUS J. VLAHAKES, MD
Professor of Surgery, Division of Cardiac
Surgery, Harvard Medical School,
Massachusetts General Hospital, Boston,
Massachusetts

Contents

> Under normal baseline conditions the unique anatomy, myocardial ultrastructure, and coronary physiology of the right ventricle (RV) reflect a high-volume low-pressure pump. Early work described the RV as a passive conduit with minimal pumping capability. It is now appreciated that through a mechanism of ventricular interdependence, RV systolic function and diastolic load are extremely important in the prognosis and treatment of congestive heart failure, cardiac transplantation, pulmonary hypertension, congenital heart disease, and left ventricle assist devices. Magnetic resonance imaging with three-dimensional analysis has shown the complex geometry of the RV and the interaction of both ventricles within the pericardium.

> For many years, the right ventricle (RV) was considered less relevant in cardiac disease than its left counterpart, partly because of limited ability to noninvasively evaluate the RV with accuracy. From an earlier period when chest x-ray and invasive contrast ventriculography were the only available imaging modalities, the development of ultrasound and nuclear techniques represented important steps forward for noninvasive RV assessment. Advances in echocardiography, computed tomography, and magnetic resonance imaging provide new insights into the anatomy and function of the RV, and its importance in health and disease. In this article, we review the current state of RV imaging.

> Underappreciated is the fact that the right ventricle is often the primary determinant of long-term morbidity and mortality in patients with congenital heart disease. Right ventricular performance in these patients depends on a unique set of physiologic and pathophysiologic factors that are rarely considered in acquired heart disease. This article explores this unique physiology and pathophysiology in the hope that it will enhance understanding of a wide variety of congenital cardiac anomalies.

> This article reviews the pathophysiology, hemodynamics, natural history, and management of patients with inferior myocardial infarction complicated by right ventricular infarction. Five key areas are highlighted in which advances may impact catheterization and laboratory management of these acutely ill patients.

It is critically important to quickly recognize and treat acute pulmonary embolism (PE). Submassive and massive PEs are associated with right ventricular (RV) dysfunction and may culminate in RV failure, cardiac arrest, and death. A rapid and coordinated diagnostic and management approach can maximize success and save lives.

Right ventricular (RV) dysfunction arises in chronic lung disease when chronic hypoxemia and disruption of pulmonary vascular beds increase ventricular afterload. RV dysfunction is defined by hypertrophy with preserved myocardial contractility and cardiac output. RV hypertrophy seems to be a common complication of chronic and advanced lung disease. RV failure is rare, except during acute exacerbations of chronic lung disease or when multiple comorbidities are present. Treatment is targeted at correcting hypoxia and improving pulmonary gas exchange and mechanics. There are no data supporting the use of pulmonary hypertension-specific therapies for patients with RV dysfunction secondary to chronic lung disease.

The right ventricle (RV) is not well suited to chronic pressure overload and often fails to adequately compensate. Mechanisms that allow the RV to respond to acute pressure overload often become maladaptive and contribute to its failure, including the effects of pulmonary hypertension on RV myocardial perfusion, the influence of interventricular dependence on RV function, and metabolic shifts in the RV myocardium from fatty acid to glycolysis. Medications to treat pulmonary hypertension have focused on pulmonary vasodilatation. Their effects on RV function may determine their effectiveness. How new medications affect right ventricular performance must be addressed.

Right ventricular physiology is characterized by its close relationship with the pulmonary circuit. The right ventricle can accommodate significant changes in preload, but is highly sensitive to increases in afterload. Progressive dilatation and dysfunction can initiate a cycle of oxygen supply-demand mismatch that ultimately leads to right ventricular failure. Echocardiography and cardiac magnetic resonance imaging are the primary modalities used for non-invasive assessment of right ventricular function. The management of right ventricular failure centers on the optimization of preload, afterload and contractility. Few targeted therapies exist, although novel agents have shown promise in early studies.

Right ventricular (RV) failure remains a major problem in cardiac surgery, particularly in the setting of heart transplantation and following institution of left ventricular support. Experimental studies have shown that RV function is derived from 2 sources: the free wall of the RV and the interventricular septum. Management of RV failure involves not only decreasing RV afterload, but also optimizing both contributions to RV function, which is best achieved by optimizing developed systemic pressure. Techniques for managing the pulmonary circulation and strategies for optimizing RV function in various clinical settings are presented.

Right ventricular (RV) failure that develops following LVAD placement is an important and challenging complication that occurs in approximately 15–25% of LVAD patients. Thus, a thorough evaluation that identifies pre-operative clinical predictors of RV failure is crucial to aid in the appropriate treatment and prognostication. Following LVAD implant, three major physiologic changes invariably occur that will influence RV function: an increase in RV preload, a decrease in RV afterload, and an alteration in RV contractility. Management strategies exist to minimize the likelihood and severity of RV failure post-LVAD. Further studies are needed that also focus on intermediate and late post-LVAD RV failure.

Right ventricular (RV) failure is an increasingly common clinical problem that may require mechanical support. In contrast to severe left ventricular failure, RV failure is typically more reversible. Therefore, application of shorter-term percutaneous support devices is potentially attractive. Current innovations promise greater availability of such percutaneous RV support devices. This article considers the available mechanical approaches to provide hemodynamic support to treat profound RV failure in the common clinical scenarios in which percutaneous mechanical RV support may be most beneficial.

Erratum

An error was made in the November 2011 issue of *Cardiology Clinics* on pages 568, 569 and 570 in "The Future of Adult Cardiac Assist Devices: Novel Systems and Mechanical Circulatory Support Strategies" by Carlo R. Bartoli and Robert D. Dowling. Procyrion Incorporated and the Procyrion circulatory assist device were spelled incorrectly. Procyrion is the correct spelling.

In addition, the credit line for Figure 7 on page 570 was erroneously given as "Courtesy of Heart-Ware Inc (Miami Lakes, FL); with permission. Courtesy of Daniel Tamez." The correct credit line for Figure 7 is "From Procyrion Inc. (Houston, TX); with permission. Courtesy of Michael Cuchiara."

CARDIOLOGY CLINICS

NOW AVAILABLE FOR YOUR iPhone and iPad

Foreword

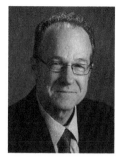

Michael H. Crawford, MD
Consulting Editor

The right ventricle is an interesting part of the heart. It is absent in invertebrates, fish, amphibians, and most reptiles, appearing in evolution in birds and mammals. The left heart and probably both atria form from the primitive heart tube of mesodermal origin. The right ventricle is derived from neural crest cells that migrate to the heart during fetal development. Thus, the dismissive observation that the right ventricle seems to be an applique on the left ventricle has some truth to it. Obviously, the right ventricle was important for full adaptation to living on land and is probably largely responsible for the ability of birds and mammals to sustain a high level of physical activity. In humans we know that surgical removal of the tricuspid valve, which markedly reduces the forward output of the right ventricle, is compatible with life, but not with sustained high-level physical activity. Also, sudden failure of the right ventricle, as occurs in right ventricular infarction, can result in systemic blood pressures too low to sustain critical organ flow. Clearly under certain circumstances the right ventricle is very important to our well-being.

This issue of *Cardiology Clinics* explores the role of the right ventricle in several clinical scenarios and details how the recognition of right ventricular dysfunction can impact management. Drs Goldstein and Rich have done an outstanding job of recruiting some of the best experts on the right ventricle to discuss these issues. The issue starts with a discussion of the unique anatomy and physiology of the right ventricle, describes techniques for imaging the right ventricle, and then delves into eight unique scenarios of right ventricular dysfunction. All physicians caring for heart disease patients need to be aware of these eight problems and how to manage them.

Michael H. Crawford, MD
Division of Cardiology, Department of Medicine
University of California
San Francisco Medical Center
505 Parnassus Avenue, Box 0124
San Francisco, CA 94143-0124, USA

E-mail address:
crawfordm@medicine.ucsf.edu

cardiology.theclinics.com

Cardiol Clin 30 (2012) ix
doi:10.1016/j.ccl.2012.04.001
0733-8651/12/$ – see front matter

Preface
Faces of Right Ventricular Failure

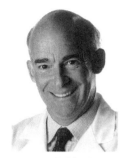 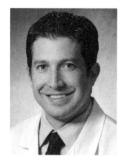

James A. Goldstein, MD   Jonathan D. Rich, MD
Guest Editors

Sir William Harvey in his 17th century treatise, *Exercitatio Anatomica de Motu Cordis et Sanguinis in Animalibus*, elucidated the circulatory system in general and provided insight into the purpose of the right ventricle (RV):

> "...as the lungs are so close at hand, and in continual motion, and the vessel that supplies them is of such dimensions, what is the use or meaning of this pulse of the right ventricle? And why was nature reduced to the necessity of adding another ventricle for the sole purpose of nourishing the lungs?"

Despite Harvey's insights four centuries ago, until relatively recently the RV was thought to be unimportant in the circulation. However, over the past three decades there has been increasing appreciation of the importance of the RV under physiologic conditions and in various disease states. In 2006, the National Heart, Lung, and Blood Institute formed a working group specifically dedicated to fostering a better understanding of RV function and failure and identifying the key areas where research efforts should be applied to advance this largely understudied field.

The Faces of RV Failure was compiled to provide a comprehensive state-of-the-art review focusing on the pathophysiology and management of RV failure in various disease states. We hope this issue will not only provide insights into the increasingly common scenarios in which RV failure complicates clinical management but also serve to stimulate physician-scientists to investigative pursuits further to move the field forward to enhance care for our patients.

James A. Goldstein, MD
Department of Cardiovascular Medicine
Beaumont Health System
3601 West 13 Mile Road
Royal Oak, MI 48073, USA

Jonathan D. Rich, MD
Section of Cardiology
Department of Medicine
University of Chicago Medical Center
5841 South Maryland Avenue
Chicago, IL 60637, USA

E-mail addresses:
JGOLDSTEIN@beaumont.edu (J.A. Goldstein)
jrich@bsd.uchicago.edu (J.D. Rich)

Cardiol Clin 30 (2012) xi
doi:10.1016/j.ccl.2012.03.013
0733-8651/12/$ – see front matter © 2012 Elsevier Inc. All rights reserved.

Anatomy and Physiology of the Right Ventricle

Louis J. Dell'Italia, MD

KEYWORDS

• Right ventricle • Anatomy • Physiology

The right ventricle (RV) because of its low-pressure working conditions and complex geometry stands in stark contrast to the left ventricle (LV). Thus, under normal baseline conditions, the unique anatomy, myocardial ultrastructure, and coronary physiology of the RV reflect a high-volume low-pressure pump. Early work by Starr[1] and others[2–4] described the RV as a passive conduit with minimal pumping capability. With improved functional imaging capabilities, it is now well appreciated that through a mechanism of ventricular interdependence, RV systolic function and diastolic load are extremely important, as is explained elsewhere in this issue, in the prognosis and treatment of congestive heart failure, cardiac transplantation, pulmonary hypertension, congenital heart disease, and LV assist devices. Magnetic resonance imaging with three-dimensional analysis has provided important insights into the complex geometry of the RV and the interaction of both ventricles within the pericardium. **Fig. 1** shows surface curvature displays of the RV and LV in a normal human individual and in a patient with left heart failure caused by mitral regurgitation and in a patient with right heart failure caused by primary pulmonary hypertension.

RV ANATOMY

The muscle mass of the RV is approximately one-sixth that of the LV, forming a crescent-shaped chamber comprising a sinus (body) and outflow tract in contrast to the ellipsoidal, concentric LV. Despite markedly different muscle mass and chamber geometry, both ventricles are bound together by spiraling muscle bundles encircling both ventricles in a complex interlacing fashion, forming a functionally single unit. The RV conus, or outflow tract, is of particular interest. The RV conus was recognized as being anatomically distinct from the main portion of the RV by Keith in 1924.[5] He showed that the bulbus cordis is present as a separate chamber distal to the common ventricle in all developing vertebrate embryos. In the LV, the bulbus disappears as development proceeds, whereas in the RV it remains to form the infundibulum or outflow tract. Armour and Randall[6] showed that the muscle fibers of the conus run in a parallel alignment from epicardium to endocardium in 9 different mammalian species including humans. In contrast, the muscle fibers of the sinus undergo a slow right-angular directional change from epicardium to endocardium and this fiber orientation is similar to that of the LV. Both sinus and conus have similar wall thicknesses; however, the conus has a mechanical advantage over the sinus because it has a smaller radius of curvature. Therefore, there exists an architectural and functional separation of the inflow and outflow tracts of the RV.

Schlesinger and colleagues[7] reported a lower incidence of occlusion in the conus artery than any other artery directly connected to the aorta. This feature, coupled with its location between the main left anterior descending and right coronary arteries, explains its functional importance in supplying collateral blood flow to these vessels with a higher incidence of occlusion.[8,9] In addition, the unique anatomic position of the conus artery arising close to the ostium or as a separate ostium generally results in preservation of systolic function of the RV outflow tract in patients with acute RV myocardial infarction, because ostial occlusions

Division of Cardiovascular Disease, Birmingham VA Medical Center, Birmingham, AL 35294, USA
E-mail address: loudell@uab.edu

Cardiol Clin 30 (2012) 167–187
doi:10.1016/j.ccl.2012.03.009
0733-8651/12/$ – see front matter © 2012 Published by Elsevier Inc.

cardiology.theclinics.com

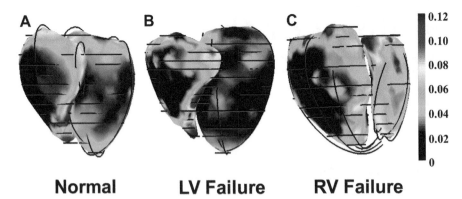

Normal   LV Failure   RV Failure

Fig. 1. Shaded surface displays of epicardial curvature in the RV and LV from a normal individuals (*A*) and from a patient with left heart failure caused by mitral regurgitation (*B*) and a patient with right heart failure caused by primary pulmonary hypertension. (*C*) These images show a commensurate increase in RV in left heart failure and the disproportionate increase in RV at the expense of LV in primary pulmonary hypertension. (*Courtesy of Drs Himanshu Gupta, Thomas Denney, and Chun Guo-Schirros.*)

of the right coronary artery are an infrequent occurrence.

Ventricular Interaction

The intimate anatomic relationship of the RV and LV, including their interlacing muscle bundles, common interatrial septum, and interventricular septum, and shared coronary blood flow, set up a continuous interplay between the 2 ventricles. Functionally, the cardiac ventricles can be viewed as 2 hydraulic pumps in series, one coupled to a highly compliant pulmonary vasculature and the other matched to a less compliant systemic circulation. Both ventricles are encased within the pericardium, which does not expand significantly in response to sudden stresses. These anatomic and functional arrangements allow for a direct as well as a series interaction when an acute or chronic hemodynamic perturbation changes the vascular load of 1 pump.

Bernheim[10] is often credited with being the first to hypothesize that alterations of 1 ventricle could affect the other. In 1910, he postulated that LV hypertrophy and dilatation could compress the RV, resulting in diminished RV function, venous congestion, and cardiac failure. Subsequently, in 1914, Henderson and Prince,[11] using an isolated cat heart preparation, showed that volume and pressure loading of 1 ventricle decreased the output and function of the contralateral ventricle. In 1956, Dexter[12] described deterioration of LV function in patients with atrial septal defects who developed RV pressure and volume overload. He called this the reverse Bernheim effect, postulating leftward septal shift with resultant impaired LV filling and function. Since these early descriptions, it has been appreciated that alterations in

compliance of 1 chamber can affect the filling of the opposite chamber. This diastolic interaction is clearly mediated by the pericardium. However, it is not the only cause of interaction because the effect is not completely abolished in the absence of the pericardium.

The pericardial sac encloses the heart and is attached to the great vessels, the sternum, the vertebral column, and the diaphragm. Consequently, it serves to hold the heart in a fixed position and to isolate and protect it from other thoracic structures. Although its presence is not essential to life, it functions to prevent the heart from acute overdistention, and its fluid lubricates the heart surface so that it can undergo motion without friction.[13] The pericardium is composed of collagen and elastin fibers embedded in a weak but viscous ground substance matrix. In the human pericardium, the collagen is arranged in 3 layers, with each layer aligned in a direction approximately 60° from the adjacent layer.[14,15] The strong collagen and relatively weak elastin fibers, as well as the viscous ground substance matrix, make the pericardium highly resistant to acute distention. Its pressure-volume and stress-strain curves are J-shaped, indicating that after an initial compliant phase, pericardial stiffness rapidly increases.[16–18] In addition, because of its layers of collagen aligned in different directions, the pericardium has uniaxial as well as biaxial stress-strain relationships, resulting in an anisotropic behavior of the pericardium. However, it has been shown in animal models that a chronic arteriovenous fistula results in an attenuation of the pericardial restraining effect over time.[19,20] This accommodation effect represents the creep and stress relaxation characteristics of the pericardium. Creep is defined as the time-dependent elongation of a material held at constant stress. Stress relaxation is the time-dependent diminution of stress held at a constant strain. These functional changes over time have been attributed to straightening of the normally wavy collagen fibers and to rearrangement of the collagen fiber geometry in the ground substance and the perpendicularly arranged elastin fibers.

From these histologic and functional studies of the pericardium, there is no question that the intact pericardium functions to restrain acute increases in volume in the intact heart. However, according to the work of Holt,[13] the initial compliant phase of the stress-strain relationship should allow physiologic increases in volume of the heart without exerting a restraining effect. However, the quantitation of this effect requires a measurement of pericardial pressure. Normal intrapericardial pressure is negative or approximately equal to zero because pericardial pressure varies with pleural pressure at the same hydrostatic level.[21] The true distending pressure of the ventricular cavity is determined by a measurement of transmural pressure, which equals cavitary pressure minus adjacent intrapericardial pressure.[22] Thus, the normally negative pericardial pressure produces a distending pressure that is higher than the cavitary pressure. However, calculation of transmural pressure in intact animals in clinical situations is complicated by the difficulties in measuring pericardial pressure.

Smiseth and colleagues[23] showed that conventional fluid-filled catheters cannot accurately measure pericardial pressure, especially at lower or minimal pericardial volume. Under normal circumstances, the pericardial cavity is a potential space and thus pericardial pressure is best described as a surface pressure rather than a liquid pressure. From the same laboratory, Smiseth and colleagues[24] and Tyberg and colleagues[25] showed that a flat, liquid-filled balloon is a more appropriate tool for accurate measurement of pericardial surface pressure, with the caveat that implementation of this method may introduce artifactual pericardial restriction caused by local distortion of the very small pericardial space.[26] Nevertheless, Tyberg and colleagues[27] measured RV and LV pericardial pressures in patients instrumented with flat, liquid-containing silastic balloons in the pericardial space during elective cardiac surgery. During progressive volume loading, RV pericardial pressure was equal to LV pericardial pressure over central venous pressures ranging from 4 to 18 mm Hg and RV late-diastolic (pre-a-wave) cavitary pressure correlated with LV pericardial pressure.

Although it is controversial whether an accurate transmural pressure can be measured in an animal

model or in the human, it can be assumed that the intact pericardium affects the measured intracavitary pressure as pericardial volume increases beyond its early compliant phase. This observation is especially applicable to the more distensible RV. This response is resisted by the pericardium beyond its unstressed volume, resulting in increase of intracavitary pressures, which does not reflect the true distending pressure or volume of the contralateral LV. This physiologic phenomenon has important clinical implications, as is discussed in the articles on acute RV infarction and pulmonary embolus.

There is evidence that pleural and mediastinal structures can also impart a restraining effect similar to the pericardium. Fewell and coworkers[28,29] reported that LV diastolic compliance can be affected by positive end-expiratory pressure with and without an intact pericardium. The mechanism of this effect may be a direct transmission of pressure to the pericardial space. However, the acute increase in pulmonary afterload may distend the right heart chambers at the expense of the left-sided chambers and cause pericardial restraint if total heart volume increases beyond the compliant phase of the pericardial pressure-volume curve. Alternatively, in the absence of the pericardium, the limits of the cardiac fossa can be restrained by the adjacent lungs, sternum, and diaphragm. The clinical importance of the pericardium in the modulation of cardiac function was recently reviewed by Tyberg.[30] However, as pointed out in this review, the effects of the pericardium on cardiac physiology were predicted by Louis Katz in 1954[31]:

Even the use of end-diastolic pressure as an index of end-diastolic volume is not justified … Furthermore, if the expansion of the heart is limited, for example by the pericardium, changes in end-diastolic pressure lose much of their meaning in terms of changes in end-diastolic volume.

Interventricular Septum

Because of its position, the interventricular septum participates in the function of both the RV and LV. However, few studies have concentrated on the functional contribution of the interventricular septum to right and left ventricular stroke output. Molaug and colleagues[32] studied myocardial cord lengths measured from piezoelectric crystals in the longitudinal axis of the interventricular septum and free walls of the RV and LV during saline infusion. End-diastolic cord lengths and myocardial shortening increased equivalent amounts in the septum and free walls of both ventricles as end-diastolic pressures increased to greater than 10 mm Hg in both ventricles. Subsequent pericardotomy further increased end-diastolic segment lengths and myocardial shortening in the septum and free walls as end-diastolic pressures decreased 1 to 2 mm Hg. In a subset of dogs, longitudinal and transverse septal dimensions responded in a similar fashion. Thus, these data support the conclusion that Frank-Starling mechanism is activated in the interventricular septum and that the increase in right and left ventricular end-diastolic pressures is not mediated by a shift in septal position but rather by the restraining effect of the pericardium during volume expansion. However, without a measure of septal curvature, the latter statement cannot be made definitively.

From the many studies of acute pulmonary hypertension in animal models, leftward shift of the interventricular septum plays an important role in the mechanism of ventricular interaction. However, the dynamics of diastolic and especially systolic septal position are not completely explained by the transseptal pressure gradient alone. This situation has been verified by the observation that the septum maintains a leftward displacement at end-systole after acute RV hypertension despite an LV pressure that exceeds RV pressure.[33,34] Piene and colleagues[33] studied the effect of the transseptal pressure gradient on the position of the interventricular septum by varying afterload and preload for both the RV and LV in the anesthetized open-chested dog. They found that the influence of the transseptal pressure gradient on the position of the interventricular septum reduced to one-tenth when changing from end-diastole to end-systole. These

investigators concluded that this finding was probably because of the relatively low wall stiffness at end-diastole, making parallel-acting forces negligible, whereas at end-systole septal position was modulated more by contractile properties of the septum itself, forces in the septal-RV free wall attachment zones, and septal geometry changes that must occur to create a force balance across the heart when the afterload on 1 side of the heart is increased acutely. These conclusions, although difficult to prove, seem plausible because the septum has a specific geometry and radius of curvature and it is composed of muscle fibers with a specific fiber orientation. Therefore, septal position is most likely determined by the combined LV and RV pressure acting in the direction parallel to the septum and oppositely in the transverse direction.

RV Chamber Characteristics

The thinner RV free wall and conus comprise a markedly different chamber geometry that has one-sixth the mass and operates at volumes slightly greater than the LV. At the chamber level, pressure-volume relationships from isolated hearts show that the RV has greater chamber distensibility than the LV. as depicted in **Fig. 2**. Because the RV and LV are composed of the same interlacing muscle fibers that encircle the heart, the greater distensibility reflects a necessary functional difference of 2 pumps in series having equal stroke outputs but coupled to markedly different vascular loads. Diastolic ventricular interaction is present on a moment-to-moment and beat-to-beat basis, especially during respiration; however, ventricular

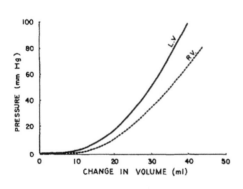
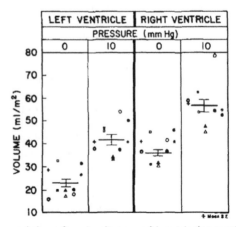

Fig. 2. Ventricular volume-pressure relationship in the normal dog after simultaneous biventricular continuous injection of Ringer solution, showing the greater distensibility of the RV compared with the LV. Ventricular volume recorded at 0 and 10 mm Hg pressure in the normal dog. Each symbol represents the average ventricular volume of an individual experiment. (*From* Laks MM, Garner D, Swan HJC. Volumes and compliances measured simultaneously in the right and left ventricles of the dog. Circ Res 1967;20:565–9; with permission.)

interaction is most apparent with acute changes in ventricular volume.

The existence of ventricular interaction can be quantified by curve fitting the diastolic pressure-volume curves of 1 ventricle as the loading conditions of the opposite ventricle are changed. Numerous studies in various animal preparations and in humans have studied the mechanism of ventricular interaction and the relative role of pericardial restraint or position of the interventricular septum in the cause of parallel shifts of the diastolic pressure-volume relationship of both ventricles under altered loading conditions.[35]

In the postmortem isolated heart preparation, Laks and colleagues[36] and Taylor and colleagues[37] reported that increased RV volume shifts the LV diastolic pressure-volume relation upward in the absence of the pericardium. In the isolated beating heart, Bemis and colleagues[38] and Santamore and colleagues[39] reported that independent loading of 1 ventricle shifted the diastolic pressure-volume relation of the contralateral ventricle upward. These investigators also reported that leftward shifting of the interventricular septum decreased chamber dimensions of the LV during RV loading. These effects were observed in the absence of the pericardium, underscoring the importance of the anatomic continuity brought about by the interventricular septum and muscle fiber arrangement of the 2 ventricles.

Subsequent studies in the isolated heart have elucidated the importance of pericardial restraint in mediating ventricular interdependence. Spadaro and colleagues[40] used an intraventricular balloon to record LV volume during progressive increases in RV filling pressure with the pericardium widely unopposed, partially closed, and completely closed. The LV diastolic pressure-volume relation was, in a leftward and parallel manner, shifted upward under each condition, but the effect was greatly augmented with the pericardium closed. Janicki and Weber[41] reported a parallel upward shift of the RV diastolic pressure-volume relation with the pericardium closed during progressive increases in LV volume using a similar preparation. Moreover, Maruyama and colleagues[42] reported that independent increases in the volume of each of the 4 cardiac chambers shifted the pressure-volume relation of the other 3 chambers upward and to the left in the postmortem isolated heart. This effect was observed with or without the pericardium but was greatly accentuated by the closed pericardium. Thus, the significance of the pericardium in modulating LV diastolic pressure-volume relationship depends on the relation of the change in volume of the heart to that of the initial unstressed volume of the pericardium. The work of Maruyama and colleagues in the isolated heart model provides some support to this contention because an independent increase in volume of any chamber shifted the LV pressure-volume curve upward and to the to the left. Although these studies in the isolated heart and other studies[43–45] report a tight coupling of the right and left ventricular diastolic pressure-volume relation, they are nonphysiologic because (1) the volume of 1 ventricle is independently increased as the other is held constant, (2) the pericardium is disturbed surgically, and (3) the ventricles are stripped of their respective arterial circulations.

VENTRICULAR INTERACTION IN THE INTACT CIRCULATION

In the anesthetized and awake preinstrumented dog, Tyberg and colleagues[46] and Shirato and colleagues[47] reported that the LV diastolic pressure-volume and pressure-dimension relation were shifted upward and to the left by volume expansion. In both of these studies, the parallel shifts of the LV diastolic pressure-volume relationship were largely absent on removal of the pericardium. Although these and other studies show the importance of the pericardium in mediating changes in the passive diastolic pressure-volume relation, Tyson and colleagues[48] have cautioned that the experimental preparation may introduce significant artifactual pericardial restriction. In their study of the preinstrumented dog, resuturing a small pericardial incision at the base of the heart produced significantly lower intrapericardial pressures when compared with a similar reapproximation of the more conventional longitudinal incision from base to apex. Consequently, these investigators concluded that the effects of the normal undisturbed pericardium may have less of an effect on diastolic filling than that reported in the preinstrumented animal.

The most striking examples of acute ventricular interaction occur in the setting of acute pulmonary embolus (**Fig. 3**), implantation of an LV assist device (**Fig. 4**), acute RV failure after cardiac transplantation, or RV myocardial infarction. In each case, the cause of low cardiac output is RV distension in the stiff pericardium, resulting in decreased LV preload. It has long been appreciated that acute severe pulmonary embolism with increased pulmonary artery and RV pressure may result in decreased cardiac output, systemic arterial hypotension, and death.[49–52] Numerous studies in animal models have reported the effects of acute pulmonary artery constriction[45,53–56] or artifactually produced pulmonary embolus[57–59] in various

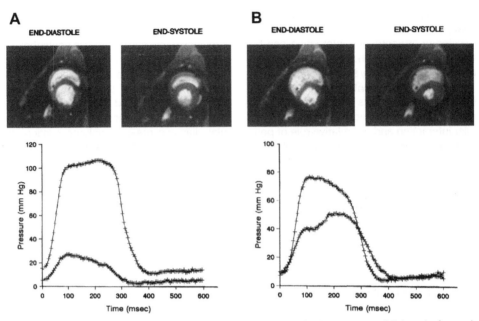

Fig. 3. Short-axis images of LV and RV at end-diastole and end-systole during control (*A*) and after pulmonary embolus (*B*). After pulmonary embolus, there is marked enlargement of RV at end-diastole and end-systole and leftward displacement of interventricular septum. (*Bottom*) Analogue to digitally converted LV and RV pressures during control and after pulmonary embolus, showing the late RV pressure wave caused by wave reflection. (*From* Dell'Italia LJ, Pearce DJ, Blackwell GG, et al. Right and left ventricular volumes and function after acute pulmonary hypertension in the intact dog. J Appl Physiol 1995;78:2320–27; with permission.)

dog models. In the animal preinstrumented with LV epicardial or endocardial sonomicrometers, acute constriction of pulmonary artery results in significant reductions in the interventricular septal to lateral wall LV dimensions in both systole and diastole, with little effect on the anteroposterior and base-apex dimensions. Furthermore, the decrease in LV +dP/dt$_{max}$ was related to the

reduction in LV preload and not to a reduction in contractility.[55] Therefore, these studies clearly show that the underfilling of the LV in acute RV pressure overload results from the anatomic contiguity of the 2 ventricles mediated by the shared interventricular septum. Furthermore, transmural LV pressure (LV end-diastolic pressure minus directly measured intrapericardial pressure) accurately

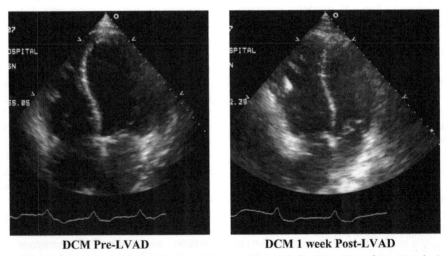

DCM Pre-LVAD   DCM 1 week Post-LVAD

Fig. 4. Four-chamber views of a patient with heart failure before and after insertion of LV assist device showing the increase in RV dimensions and decrease in LV dimensions as a result of the unloading effect of the LV assist device. (*Courtesy of* Dr Sumanth Prabhu.)

reflected the significant changes in LV dimensions.[58] Thus, when pericardial restraint and ventricular inter-action are taken into account, neither compliance nor contractility is significantly affected and reduced performance results primarily from impaired LV dia-stolic filling. As reported in the article on RV myocar-dial infarction, opening of the pericardium after acute pulmonary hypertension increased LV size and improved cardiac output by 35%, showing the importance of the restraining effects of pericardium and leftward septal shifting with acute increases in RV afterload (**Fig. 5**).[59]

The potential mechanism(s) responsible for parallel shifts in the diastolic pressure-volume rela-tion in response to acute alterations in loading include changes in intrinsic myocardial factors or external constraints on the ventricular chambers. Variations in intrinsic chamber properties are highly unlikely because multiple investigations have shown this phenomenon with interventions and pharmacologic agents that are devoid of direct myocardial effects. Extrinsic factors including pleural pressure, pericardial restraint, and ventricular interaction mediated through shift-ing of the interventricular septum may produce acute parallel shifts in the ventricular diastolic pressure-volume relation. The mechanism of ventricular interaction is difficult to evaluate in the conscious human because of the inability to accu-rately measure simultaneous right and left ventric-ular volumes. Ludbrook and colleagues[60] have shown the importance of RV filling pressure in

determining the LV diastolic pressure-volume relation. In this study, amyl nitrite caused no down-ward displacement of the LV diastolic pressure-volume relation when compared with nitroglycerin, which produced a similar reduction in mean arte-rial pressure but shifted the pressure-volume rela-tion downward. This phenomenon was attributed to the failure of amyl nitrate to decrease RV dia-stolic pressure in contrast to the significant decrease in RV filling pressure resulting from nitro-glycerin infusion. In another human study, an increase in total systemic peripheral resistance imposed an acute increase in afterload on the LV and RV and, through a mechanism of ventricular interaction, resulted in a parallel upward shift of the RV diastolic pressure-volume relationship (**Fig. 6**).[61] Analysis of biplane orthogonal regional RV end-diastolic dimensions revealed that resul-tant increased volumes were largely mediated by lengthening of the distance between the septum and the RV free wall. This finding suggests that the restraining effect of the pericardium rather than shifting of the interventricular septum is mostly responsible for the parallel upward shift of the RV diastolic pressure-volume relation. In the intact circulation, when acute alterations in arterial and venous pressures affect all 4 heart chambers simultaneously and total cardiac volume is varied, pericardial restraint rather than shifting of the interventricular septum may be the predominant mechanism mediating these changes in passive diastolic properties of the ventricles.

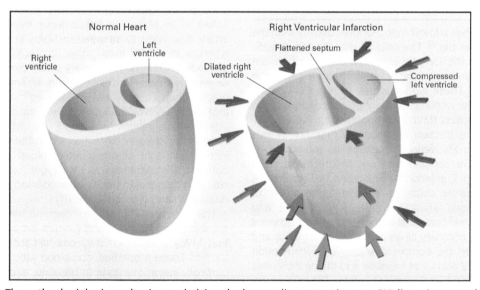

Fig. 5. The pathophysiologic mechanism underlying the low cardiac output in acute RV distension caused by RV infarction or acute pulmonary embolus. The low-output state is mediated by ventricular interaction (resulting in a flattened septum) and the restraining effect of the pericardium (*arrows*) during acute RV distention. (*From* Dell'Italia LJ. Reperfusion for right ventricular myocardial infarction. N Eng J Med 1998;338:978–80; with permis-sion. Copyright © 1998 Massachusetts Medical Society.)

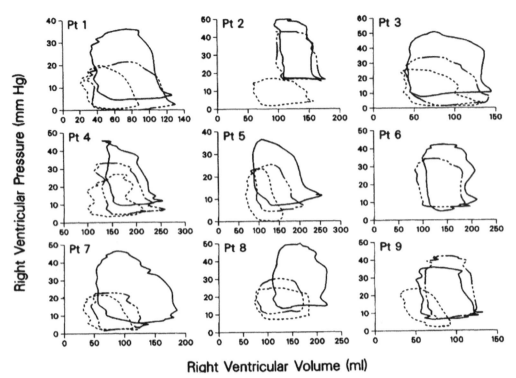

Right Ventricular Volume (ml)

Fig. 6. RV pressure-volume loops for 9 study patients having simultaneous high-fidelity RV pressures and RV biplane cineangiography, showing a parallel upward shift of the RV diastolic pressure-volume relation with changes in RV loading achieved with nitroprusside and phenylephrine. dotted line, low (nitroprusside); dashed dotted line, medium; solid line, high (phenylephrine). (*From* Dell'Italia LJ, Walsh RA. Right ventricular diastolic pressure-volume relations and regional dimensions during acute alterations in loading conditions. Circulation 1988;77:1276–82; with permission.)

RV Myocardial Ultrastructure, Oxygen Demand, and Biochemistry

The RV has a lower mitochondrial density than the LV of the pig.[62] The ratio of mitochondria/myofibrils of the LV and interventricular septum are similar and significantly greater than the ratios in the RV. These higher values for the LV indicate its greater workload and higher myocardial oxygen consumption (MVo_2) compared with the RV. RV oxygen extraction is difficult to measure in vivo because RV venous drainage is accomplished through a complex network of Thebesian veins and 5 to 7 anterior cardiac veins.[63] Therefore, it is difficult to obtain an accurate assessment of the venous efflux from the RV. Kasachi and colleagues[64] cannulated the anterior cardiac veins and the coronary sinus in 5 open-chest dogs and examined the comparative oxygen consumption of the RV and LV at baseline and during increases in afterload and inotropic state. RV MVo_2 was approximately one-half that of the LV (4.0 + 0.3 vs 8.6 + 1.4 mL O_2/min/100 g) and right coronary artery blood flow was lower than coronary blood flow in the left anterior descending artery (46 + 3

vs 87 + 5 mL/min/g) under baseline conditions. Pacing, isoproterenol, and methoxamine stress resulted in increases in left anterior descending artery flow with no increase in MVo_2 in the LV, whereas in the RV these stresses resulted in an increase in both right coronary artery blood flow as well as oxygen extraction. In a similar animal preparation, Takeda and colleagues[65] showed that acute RV volume loading by creation of an arteriovenous shunt increased RV MVo_2 by augmented oxygen extraction in addition to an increase in right coronary artery blood flow. In contrast, the increment in LV oxygen extraction was less than that in the RV after opening an arterioatrial shunt (31 vs 54%, $P<.01$).

The reduced RV oxygen demand results in a lower blood flow rate and oxygen extraction so that MVo_2 is approximately one-half that of the LV.[66,67] These properties, combined with a higher coronary vasomotor tone at baseline, explain the unique ability of the RV to increase oxygen extraction in response to afterload and inotropic stress and to sustain coronary occlusion for greater than twice the time than the left coronary artery to achieve one-half peak reactive hyperemia.

However, these properties were abolished in dogs with RV hypertrophy caused by pulmonary artery banding, resulting in responses that were indistinguishable from those of the LV.[68]

The RV with its thinner wall and lower operating pressures offers other interesting contrasts regarding coronary flow dynamics throughout the cardiac cycle, resulting in a systolic/diastolic flow ratio that is greater in coronary vessels that perfuse the RV than the LV.[69–75] Normal phasic flow in the right and left coronary arteries has been extensively studied in the dog using electromagnetic flow probes. This is a unique preparation because the canine right coronary artery is a nondominant vessel, which supplies only the RV free wall. Systolic coronary artery flow commences rapidly in both arteries after opening of the aortic valves, producing an early peak, which declines immediately to a higher plateau throughout systole in the right coronary artery when compared with the left coronary artery. Subsequently, the level of flow in the right coronary artery during diastole remains relatively constant in contrast to the rapidly declining diastolic flow in the left coronary circulation. Lowensohn and colleagues[75] reported a systolic/diastolic flow ratio of 36% + 1.3% in the right coronary artery and a substantially lower ratio of 13% + 3.6% in the left circumflex artery of the conscious dog. However, systolic flow was markedly reduced and was inversely related to peak RV systolic pressure in dogs with congenital pulmonic stenosis.

It seems that the low oxygen demands of the RV may represent the most important factor in protecting its myocardium from irreversible ischemic damage after right coronary occlusion. The ability to extract more oxygen during times of stress in addition to both systolic and diastolic coronary flow provides a greater reserve of nutrients and oxygen during ischemia. All of these factors may work in concert to prevent irreversible ischemic damage to the RV. A sparing of RV necrosis was found in the farm pig after right coronary occlusion without an extensive network of collateral vessel development.[76] However, preexisting RV hypertrophy induced by pulmonary artery banding resulted in RV necrosis in all animals despite a similar amount of collateral vessel development in the normal and hypertrophied RVs.

Protection from ischemic damage may also explain the importance of the RV in predicting, exercise capacity, response to biventricular pacing, and morbidity and mortality in systolic heart failure. Recently, Meyer and colleagues[77] reported that in patients with advanced systolic heart failure, RV ejection fraction (RVEF) impairment is common and is associated with poor outcomes. RVEF less than 40% is a marker of increased risk of death and hospitalization, and RVEF less than 20% is an independent predictor of increased risk of death and hospitalization because of heart failure.

Another important major difference in RV and LV is that the RV inotropic response to α_1 adrenergic receptors (α_1-ARs) is switched from negative in normal to positive in heart failure RVs, through a pathway involving increased myofilament Ca^{2+} sensitivity.[78,79] α_1-ARs mediate a positive inotropic response in the mouse neonatal RV myocardium, in contrast to a negative inotropic response in the nonfailing adult RV myocardium (**Fig. 7**).[80] In

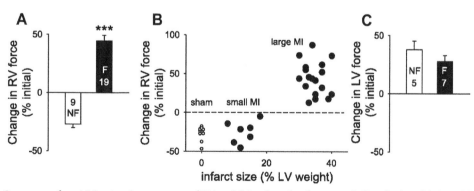

Fig. 7. Summary of α_1-AR inotropic responses of RV and LV trabeculae from nonfailing (NF) and failing (F) hearts. Inotropic responses are shown as the change of developed force induced by phenylephrine (PE) expressed relative to the developed force before PE (%initial). (A) Switch in the RV α_1-AR inotropic response from negative (in NF hearts) to positive in heart failure. (B) RV α_1-AR inotropic responses were not switched for hearts subjected to small infarcts (scar weight <20% LV weight). (C) No switch in the LV α_1-AR inotropic response in heart failure. Numbers in bars are numbers of hearts per group. ***$P<.001$. (*From* Wang G-Y, Yeh C-C, Hensen BC, et al. Heart failure switches the RV $\alpha1$-adrenergic inotropic response from negative to positive. Am J Physiol 2010;298: H213–20; with permission.)

addition, α_{1A}-AR and α_{1b}-AR density is not down-regulated in the failing LV, and α_{1A}-AR shows similar distribution and function in the human and mouse heart.[81] Increased α_1-AR inotropic responses in the RV myocardium may be an adaptive response to increased pulmonary pressures. Thus, α agonists may represent a pharmacologic target in the treatment of right heart failure.

Properties of the Pulmonary Vascular Bed

The force opposing the shortening of muscle fibers, or afterload, is a major determinant of myocardial performance in isolated muscle preparations and intact heart. Pulmonary impedance is a measure of the opposition to pulmonary artery flow. Compared with pulmonary vascular resistance, it is a more accurate measure of afterload in pulmonary circulation. The pulmonary impedance modulus has the same units as resistance but in addition it also has a term that describes the opposition to and energy cost of pulsations in the pulmonary vascular bed.[82–84] Impedance is frequency dependent and is modulated by (1) heart rate, (2) vessel stiffness or viscoelastic properties of the vessel, and (3) wave reflections. The changes in impedance resulting from large-artery stiffening or remodeling alone can markedly alter the load on the RV and can occur in the absence of a change in pulmonary vascular resistance. Pulmonary impedance in turn is closely coupled to ventricular geometry, function, and chamber pressures.[85]

Pulmonary input impedance measurements in normal animals[86–88] and man[83,89–91] have consistently shown a pulse wave velocity that was approximately one-half that of the normal systemic circulation. This situation causes reflected pressure waves to return later, after pulmonic valve closure, and seems to offset the shorter distances to reflecting sites in the pulmonary arteries so that the RV and LV are optimally matched at physiologic heart rates. These properties of the pulmonary vascular bed produce RV contractile characteristics that are different from the LV, which is coupled to a systemic circuit having a higher pressure, significantly less distensibility, and greater wave reflection. Elzinga and colleagues[92,93] and Piene[85] developed an isolated cat heart model in which the resistive and compliant components could be changed independently and related to stroke output of the ventricle. These studies showed that decreased compliance (increased characteristic impedance) and increased resistance produced equivalent decreases in left and right ventricular stroke volume. There was a striking similarity of the wave forms of pressure and flow for the RV and LV under different loading conditions. This finding strongly suggests that the 2 ventricles have comparable characteristics as pumps.

Fig. 8 shows simultaneous electrocardiogram, the first derivative of RV pressure development (dP/dt), pulmonary artery flow velocity, and high-fidelity RV and pulmonary artery pressures in a normal individual.[94–96] The normal RV pressure wave form has a low peak pressure, which occurs early in systole and subsequently decreases rapidly. The pre-ejection period and RV ejection time aid in showing minimal isovolumic contraction because of the low pulmonary artery diastolic pressure and ejection of blood as RV pressure is rapidly declining. The observation of continued forward flow in the presence of not only a declining pressure but also a negative pressure gradient emphasizes the inability of pressure measurements alone to define the mechanisms of

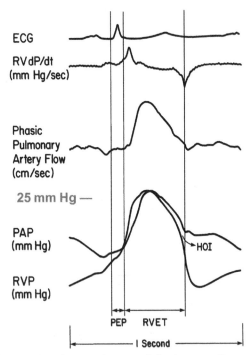

Fig. 8. Simultaneously recorded electrocardiogram (ECG), RV analogue signal of pressure development (dP/dt), phasic pulmonary artery flow, pulmonary artery pressure (PAP), and RV pressure (RVP) in a human. Vertical lines show the pre-ejection period (PEP) and RV ejection time (RVET). The hangout interval (HOI) represents the time interval between the pulmonary incisura and the RV pressure wave form, caused by ejection into the compliant pulmonary vasculature. (*From* Dell'Italia LJ, Walsh RA. Determinants of the hangout interval in response to acute alteration in pulmonary arterial pressure. Am Heart J 1988;116:1289–97; with permission.)

RV-pulmonary artery coupling because total RV afterload is composed of resistive, capacitative, inertial, and pulse wave reflection properties of the pulmonary vasculature.

The rate of pressure increase in the LV cavity is dependent on the end-diastolic pressure, peak systolic pressure, and the time spent in the development of pressure.[97,98] For all of these reasons, LV + dP/dt$_{max}$ is significantly higher than the normal RV + dP/dt$_{max}$ matched to the highly compliant pulmonary vascular bed. However, this relationship may change in response to an acute or chronic increase in afterload. **Fig. 9** shows the acute increases in RV + dP/dt$_{max}$ during intravenous phenylephrine infusion, producing progressive increases in pulmonary pressure in a normal individual.[96] At higher systolic pressure, there is an increase in duration of the isovolumic contraction phase and an increase in end-diastolic pressure, resulting in a higher peak positive dP/dt$_{max}$. In normal individuals and in patients with chronic pulmonary hypertension, there is a linear relationship between pulmonary artery pressure and peak +dP/dt$_{max}$.[99] Furthermore, high +RV dP/dt$_{max}$ values have been noted in patients with pulmonary hypertension despite clinical evidence of RV failure manifested by markedly increased right heart filling pressures, ascites, and peripheral edema.[100] Therefore, values in the normal RV are low (100–250 mm Hg/s) and do not provide a reliable index of contractility because of the load dependency of peak + dP/dt$_{max}$.

Because of a higher afterload, earlier reflection of pressure waves produces a more rounded LV pressure wave form with cessation of forward flow soon after peak pressure. The continuation of forward blood flow in the presence of a rapidly declining pressure characterizes RV ejection dynamics in the presence of normal pulmonary vasculature. However, acute and chronic RV hypertension in humans shows pressure and flow characteristics similar to those of the LV and aorta. The RV pressure-flow characteristics now resemble LV pressure-flow dynamics when a normal human individual is subjected to acute increases in afterload with phenylephrine infusion. **Fig. 9** shows that the RV pressure wave takes on the late peak from earlier wave reflection in the last one-third of systole.[96] These changes in the pulmonary vasculature also explain the termination of ejection shortly after peak pressure at high pressure loading.

The comparative configurations of pressure and flow in the pulmonary and systemic circulations

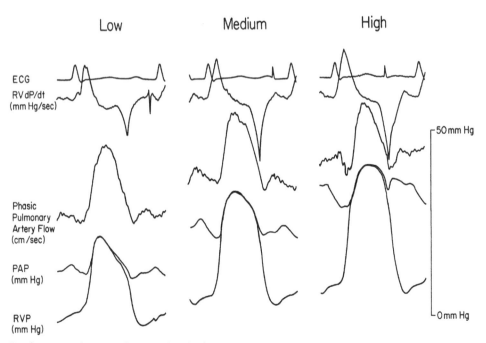

Fig. 9. Simultaneous electrocardiogram (ECG), RV dP/dt, phasic pulmonary artery (PA) flow velocity, and PA and RV pressure at low, medium, and high loading conditions produced by nitroprusside and phenylephrine infusion. The increase in RV pressure is accompanied by a higher dP/dt, greater wave reflection, and increased isovolumic contraction time. (*From* Dell'Italia LJ, Walsh RA. Application of a time varying elastance model and other end-systolic pressure-volume relations to right ventricular performance in man. Cardiovasc Res 1998;22:864–74; with permission.)

were studied by van den Boss and Westerhof[86] in the intact dog under altered loading conditions. **Fig. 10** shows the similarity of the pressure and flow pulses in the pulmonary artery and the disparity of pressure and flow pulses in the aorta, with wave reflection in large part accounting for the dissimilarity in flow and pressure in the pulmonary and systemic circulation. Consequently, the more the forward pressure wave was reflected, as in the systemic circulation, the less the measured flow resembled measured pressure wave forms. In contrast, there was significantly less wave reflection in the compliant pulmonary bed and pressure and flow resembled each other. However, serotonin infusion increased pulmonary vascular resistance and wave reflection, resulting in disparate pulmonary pressure and flow pulses, whereas in the systemic arterial circulation, nitroprusside infusion decreased total systemic resistance and wave reflection, producing more similar aortic pressure and flow wave forms. The conclusion from the studies mentioned earlier in animal models and in humans is that the differences in the normal pressure and flow patterns in the pulmonary and systemic vascular beds can be largely attributed to the highly compliant pulmonary vasculature.

Piene and Covell[101] measured RV wall force directly by using a modified Feigl auxotonic force gauge. This direct measurement of force showed the same configuration and timing as the RV pressure wave form over a wide range of cardiac outputs (**Fig. 11**). Furthermore, the force versus time plot was similar to that normally encountered in the LV. These data combined with the documented substantially lower myocardial oxygen demand and oxygen extraction when compared with that of the LV provide further supportive evidence of an optimal match of the RV and its vascular load in the normal state. However, vascular impedance measurements do not provide information regarding the load at the myocardial level, which is determined by wall thickness, chamber geometry, and pressure.

Mechanism of RV Ejection

Ejection of blood from the RV chamber emanates from an interaction of 3 different sources: free wall, interventricular septum, and conus. The conus, with its circumorally arranged muscle fibers,[6] contracts 30 to 50 milliseconds after the base and apex of the free wall.[102–104] This temporal disparity of contraction can be exaggerated by vagal stimulation or abolished by sympathetic stimulation.[105,106] The free wall contracts in a peristalsis wavelike fashion starting at the base and progressing to the apex. The decrease in surface area of the free wall shortens the base to apex dimension and decreases the septal to free wall dimension as the septum thickens toward the free wall. Using implanted sonomicrometer crystals in the RV free wall, conus, and RV septum in an open-chest canine model, Pouleur and colleagues[107] and Noble[108] showed that RV free wall and outflow tract segments had ceased

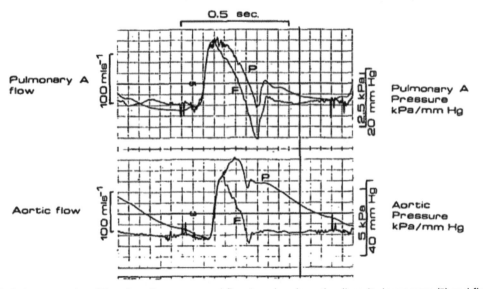

Fig. 10. Pulmonary artery (A) and aortic pressure and flow in a dog show the disparity in pressure (P) and flow (F) pulses in the pulmonary artery and aorta. (*From* van den Bos GC, Westerhof N, Randall OS. Pulse wave reflection: can it explain the differences between systemic and pulmonary pressure and flow waves? A study in dogs. Circ Res 1982;51:479–85; with permission.)

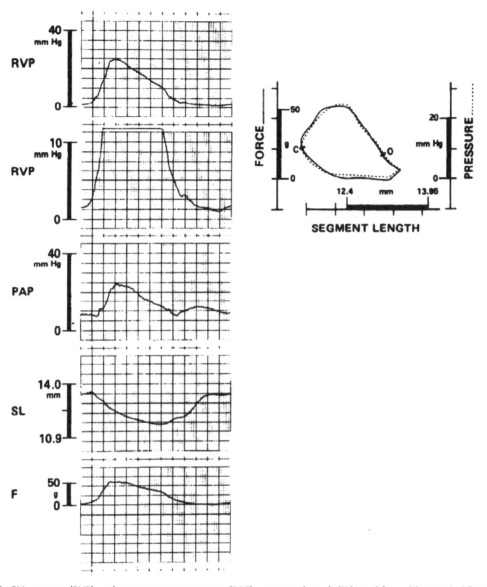

Fig. 11. RV pressure (RVP), pulmonary artery pressure (PAP), segment length (SL), and force (F) recorded from the free wall of the RV in 10 anesthetized dogs. In the right-hand panel, a force segment length and pressure segment length loop is shown. The time course of RV force (*bottom left-hand panel*) coincides closely with that of the contour of the RV wave form. In addition, the force segment length loop also coincides with the pressure segment length loop. (*From* Piene H, Covell JW. Local auxotonic systolic force and work in canine right ventricular free wall. Am J Physiol 1983;244:H186–93; with permission.)

shortening, and even lengthened, because ejection continued when RV pressure was decreasing rapidly during relaxation (**Fig. 12**). Thus, it has been proposed that RV systolic ejection dynamics is dependent on early active shortening free wall surface area and septal to free wall distance and later when the column of blood located in the outflow tract continues to flow into the pulmonary artery because of blood momentum.[109] Raizada and Covell[110] studied shortening of the outflow and inflow segments, which they called the hoop axis, as well as apex to base and free wall to septum in an open-chested dog. As in the study by Pouleur and colleagues, the shortening of the RV free wall in the hoop axis ceased before the end of pulmonary artery flow. RV free wall segments in the apex to base and free wall to septum shortened for a longer duration and their maximal excursion corresponded to zero pulmonary artery flow. However, these studies showed

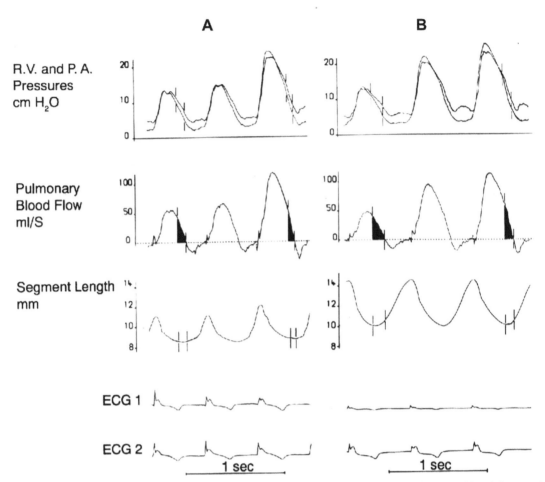

Fig. 12. (*A*) Changes in RV outflow tract pressure, pulmonary artery (PA) pressure, pulmonary blood flow, and outflow tract segment length during release of an inferior vena cava occlusion under controlled conditions. The first vertical bars on the pressure, flow, and segment length tracings identify the end of systole. The second vertical bars show the pulmonic valve closure. The shaded areas under the flow tracings show forward flow occurring during RV pressure decline. (*B*) Similar data in the inflow tract of the RV free wall, showing the presence of forward flow (*shaded area*) as segment lengths are increasing. (*From* Pouleur H, Lefèvre J, Mechelen HV, et al. Free-wall shortening and relaxation during ejection in the canine right ventricle. Am J Physiol 1980;239:H601–13; with permission.)

that RV free wall shortening ceases before the free wall to septal dimension reaches maximal excursion, suggesting a late substantial contribution of the interventricular septum to RV ejection.

Right and Left Ventricular Systolic Interaction

Following the work of Starr and colleagues,[1] subsequent experiments[2–4] showed that massive damage to the RV free wall caused little observable decrease in RV function in open pericardial dog models. These studies suggested that LV contraction contributed directly to RV systolic function.[35] Hemodynamic evidence of systolic ventricular interdependence in the anesthetized dog[111] and human[112] was also suggested by the

analogue RV dP/dt tracing, which is characteristically a broad or double-peaked signal, with one of the peaks corresponding in time to LV dP/dt$_{max}$ (**Fig. 13**). These separate components of RV and LV pressure development were accentuated during pacing from either ventricle and in individuals with ventricular asynchrony manifested by right or left bundle branch block.[112] Although these studies show that a transmission of LV developed pressure to the RV, they provide no insight into the magnitude of LV assistance.

Elzinga and colleagues[93] reported uniformly increased RV pump function graphs (RV pressure/RV output) in the presence of LV afterloaded isovolumic contractions when compared with similar graphs obtained during unloaded LV contraction.

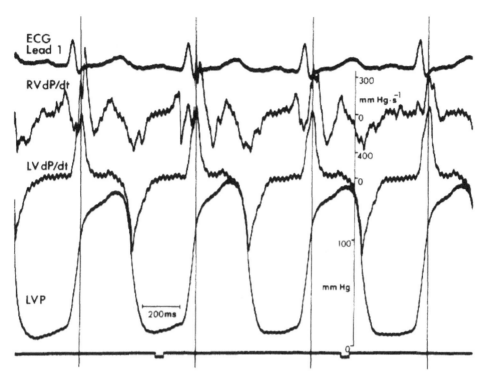

Fig. 13. RV dP/dt and LV dP/dt recorded simultaneously from an individual with incomplete right bundle branch block. Two narrowly separated RV dP/dt peaks are apparent, the first being coincident with the single LV dP/dt peak, consistent with the contribution of LV contraction to RV pressure development. (*From* Fenely MP, Gavaghan TP, Baron DW, et al. Contribution of left ventricular contraction to the generation of right ventricular systolic pressure in the human heart. Circulation 1985;71:473–80; with permission.)

In the isolated rabbit heart, Santamore and colleagues[39] showed an immediate increase in RV pressure after an increase in LV volume. Langille and Jones[113] showed an increase in RV systolic pressure and RV dP/dt in response to sudden aortic constriction in the open-chest rabbit preparation. Conversely, LV free wall ischemia produced by coronary ligation resulted in a rapid decrease in RV developed pressure in the isolated rabbit heart.[39] Although complete surgical exclusion of the RV cannot sustain life in the experimental animal,[114–117] extensive damage of the RV free wall or surgical replacement of the RV free wall with a patch[118–120] still maintains circulatory stability. Sawatini and colleagues[118] reported that the RV free wall patch moved toward the interventricular septum during systole, thereby reducing RV volume. The results of these studies suggest that the LV or the interventricular septum may assist RV function in the absence of RV free wall contraction. However, the experimental conditions of these studies are not physiologic because the pericardium is not intact and significant diastolic interaction is negated. Further studies in an intact animal preparation are required to determine the relative contribution of the LV to RV systolic performance.

The contribution of LV contraction to RV systolic performance has been appreciated in the clinical arena by the recognition of new-onset RV failure after institution of LV bypass in humans[121] and in animal models.[122,123] In a canine model of incremental LV bypass with controlled RV preload, RV dP/dt decreased significantly with maximal LV decompression.[122] The decision to use univentricular versus biventricular support is one of the key problems in the successful application in mechanical circulatory support for the treatment of patients with heart failure. The mechanisms of diastolic and systolic ventricular interaction weigh heavily in this decision and seem to depend on the pulmonary vascular load and the status of RV function in each individual case. A further discussion of other clinical implications of ventricular interaction is developed in the article on mechanical assist devices.

Right Ventricular End-systolic Pressure-Volume Relation

The RV pressure/flow characteristics determined by the highly compliant pulmonary vasculature are also reflected in its pressure-volume loop.

Dell'-Italia and Walsh[96] used simultaneous high-fidelity pressure and biplane cineventriculographic volumes to construct RV pressure-volume loops in normal individuals. **Fig. 14** shows the differences between RV and LV pressure-volume using pharmacologic interventions to achieve low, medium, and high loading. Comparison of right and left ventricular pressure-volume loops at low load shows a decreased isovolumic contraction period for both the LV with nitroprusside and the RV at baseline normal load. In addition, at end-systole (upper left corner), blood is ejected as pressure is declining in both ventricles but to a greater extent in the normal RV-pulmonary circuit compared with the LV under the influence of nitroprusside infusion. A high load shows RV and LV both have an isovolumic contraction phase and little volume decrease at end-systole as pressure declines. Thus, the pressure-volume relationship of both the RV and LV depict each ventricle ejecting into its respective arterial load at baseline and during alterations in afterload.

Ventricular contractility can be defined by the relation of instantaneous ventricular pressure, P(t), to instantaneous volume, V(t), during systole according to the equation:

$$P(t) = E(t)\,[V(t)\text{-}V_0]$$

where E(t) represents the time-varying volume elastance of the ventricle and V_0 the unstressed ventricular volume.[124,125] The equation predicts that ventricular pressure is at all instances (t) proportional to volume, the slope of the line increasing from a low value at diastole to its highest value (E_{max}) at end-systole. The slope of this relationship was highly linear for the LV and increased in response to positive inotropic therapy. Maughan and colleagues[126] were the first to show that RV performance may be described by a time-varying elastance in the isolated canine heart. Ventricular volume was measured using a water-filled latex balloon within the RV, and high-fidelity pressure using a micromanometer mounted within the balloon. Subsequently, Dell'Italia and Walsh[96] studied RV chamber mechanics in normal human individuals using cast-validated biplane cineventriculographic volumes and high-fidelity pressure measurements. The results of this study showed that RV systolic function could be approximated using a time-varying elastance model (**Fig. 15**). However, the RV showed important quantitative differences compared with the LV, manifested by lower slope values and higher V_0 values. These findings are most likely explained by the lower RV operating pressures, larger volumes, and reduced mass. Work in humans by Brown and colleagues[127] reported similar findings

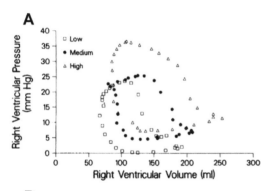

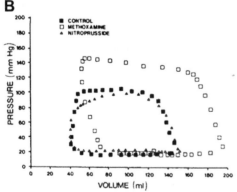

Fig. 14. RV pressure-volume loops (*upper panel A*) and LV pressure-volume loops (*lower panel B*) at low, medium, and high loading conditions, showing the differences in RV and LV ejection dynamics at low load and their similarity at higher load. (*From* Dell'Italia LJ, Santamore WP. Can indices of left ventricular function be applied to the right ventricle? The right heart. Prog Cardiovasc Dis 1998;40:309–24; with permission.)

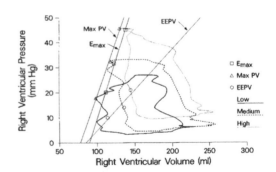

Fig. 15. The slopes of maximum time-varying elastance (E_{max}), maximum pressure/volume ratio (maxPV), and end ejection pressure/volume (EEPV) are displayed for the RV by lines of best fit by passing through 3 points of each pressure-volume loop. (*From* Dell'Italia LJ, Walsh RA. Application of a time varying elastance model and other end-systolic pressure-volume relations to right ventricular performance in man. Cardiovasc Res 1998;22:864–74; with permission.)

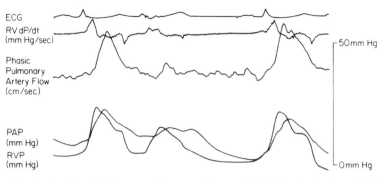

Fig. 16. Analogue signals showing simultaneous electrocardiogram (ECG) first derivative of right ventricular (RV) dp/dt, phasic pulmonary artery flow, high-fidelity pulmonary artery pressure (PAP and RVP) during the control and postextrasystolic potentiation beat in a normal individual. RV + dP/dt decreases despite an increase in stroke volume in the postextrasystolic contraction caused by the lack of isovolumic contraction. (*From* Dell'Italia LJ. Mechanism of post extrasystolic potentiation in the RV in man. Am J Cardiol 1990;65:736–41; with permission.)

using simultaneous high-fidelity RV pressure and radionuclide ventriculographic-derived volumes. In addition, studies in the isolated heart[126] and in humans[127] showed that the slope of the RV end-systolic pressure-volume relationship increases in response to inotropic stress. Therefore, the RV follows the construct of time-varying elastance, thereby suggesting that the RV and LV behave as hydraulic pumps optimally matched to their respective arterial loads.

Peak chamber elastance is obtained by the maximum slope of the linear regression applied to multiple isochronal, simultaneous pressure-volume points derived during altered loading conditions. In an attempt to simplify the quantification of chamber elastance for clinical use, time-independent pressure-volume relations near end-systole, such as the maximum pressure/volume ratio, end ejection (dicrotic notch) pressure/volume, or peak pressure/minimum volume, have been used to construct end-systolic pressure-volume relations. In the LV, the slopes obtained from these measures of end-systole correlate with E_{max}[128] because end ejection has a close temporal relation to the point of peak systolic elastance.[129] However, RV ejection proceeds beyond the points of peak pressure and peak systolic elastance because of greater pulmonary arterial compliance. RV end-systolic pressure-volume relations near end ejection (dicrotic notch/minimum volume) and peak pressure/minimum volume underestimate E(t) because of the wide temporal separation between peak systolic elastance and end ejection in the RV. However, the slopes derived from the maximum pressure/volume ratio correlated with E_{max} both at rest and after positive inotropic stimulation. Therefore, this marker of end-systole could be used in clinical studies in which the end-systolic

pressure-volume relationship is used as a means to describe pump performance of the RV.

Force-Interval Relation

The force-interval relation has been studied extensively in the LV of humans[130–132] and in the isolated heart,[133] showing that after longer filling periods, stroke volume is increased above baseline. Despite the marked differences in geometry, architecture, and muscle mass, the RV follows the force-interval relationship in the isolated heart in which volume was recorded from an intraventricular balloon.[134] Dell'Italia studied postextrasystolic potentiation in the RV of human individuals comparing 16 sinus beats and postextrasystolic beats during simultaneous right ventricular cineangiography and high-fidelity pressure monitoring.[135] Postextrasystolic beats had an average 22% increase in cycle length. In the postextrasystolic beat the end-diastolic pressure, end-diastolic volume, stroke volume, and ejection fraction increased significantly. However, as opposed to the LV, RV + dP/dt_{max} did not change because RV dP/dt_{max} has a shortened isovolumic contraction and decreased developed pressure (pulmonary artery diastolic minus right ventricular end-diastolic pressure), as shown in **Fig. 16**. This response further underscores the inability of RV dP/dt_{max} as a measure of RV contractility.

REFERENCES

1. Starr I, Jeffers WA, Meade RH. The absence of conspicuous increments of venous pressure after severe damage to the right ventricle of the dog, with a discussion of the relation between clinical congestive failure and heart disease. Am Heart J 1943;26:291–301.

2. Bakos AC. The question of the function of the right ventricular myocardium: an experimental study. Circulation 1950;1:724–31.

3. Kagan A. Dynamic responses of the right ventricle following extensive damage by cauterization. Circulation 1952;5:816–23.

4. Donald DE, Essex HE. Pressure studies after inactivation of the major portion of the canine right ventricle. Am J Physiol 1954;176:155–61.

5. Keith A. Fate of the bulbus cordis in the human heart. Lancet 1924;2:1267–73.

6. Armour JA, Randall WC. Structural basis for cardiac function. Am J Physiol 1970;218(6):1517–23.

7. Schlesinger MJ, Zoll PN, Wessler S. The conus artery: a third coronary artery. Am Heart J 1949; 38:823–36.

8. Levin DC, Beckmann CF, Garnic JD, et al. Frequency and clinical significance of failure to visualize the conus artery during coronary arteriography. Circulation 1981;63(4):833–7.

9. Adams J, Treasure T. Variable anatomy of the right coronary artery supply to the left ventricle. Thorax 1985;40:618–20.

10. Bernheim D. De l'asystolie veineuse dans l'hypertrophie du coeur gauche par stenose concomitante du ventricule droit. Rev Med 1910;39:785.

11. Henderson Y, Prince AL. The relative systolic discharges of the right and left ventricles and their bearing on pulmonary congestion and depletion. Heart 1914;5:217–26.

12. Dexter L. Atrial septal defect. Br Heart J 1956;18: 209–25.

13. Holt JP. The normal pericardium. Am J Cardiol 1970;26:455–65.

14. Elias H, Boyd LJ. Notes on the anatomy, embryology, and histology of the pericardium. N Y Med Coll News Notes 1960;2:50–75.

15. Ishira T, Ferrans VJ, Jones M, et al. Histological and ultrastructural features of normal and human parietal pericardium. Am J Cardiol 1980;46: 744–53.

16. Lee JM, Boughner DR. Tissue mechanics of canine pericardium in different test environments. Circ Res 1981;49:533–44.

17. Weigner AW, Bing OHL, Borg TK, et al. Mechanical and structural correlates of canine pericardium. Circ Res 1981;49:807–14.

18. Holt JP, Rhode EA, Kines H. Pericardial and ventricular pressure. Circ Res 1960;8:1171–81.

19. Freeman GL, LeWinter MM. Pericardial adaptations during chronic cardiac dilatation in dogs. Circ Res 1984;54:294–300.

20. LeWinter MM, Pavelec R. Influence of the pericardium on left ventricular end-diastolic pressure-segment relations during early and later stages of experimental chronic volume overload in dogs. Circ Res 1982;50:501–9.

21. Shabetai R. The pericardium: an essay on some recent developments. Am J Cardiol 1978;42: 1036–43.

22. Spodick DH. The normal and diseased pericardium: current concepts of pericardial physiology, diagnosis and treatment. J Am Coll Cardiol 1983;1:240–51.

23. Smiseth OA, Frais MA, Kingma I, et al. Assessment of pericardial restraint in dogs. Circulation 1985;71: 158–64.

24. Smiseth OA, Refsum H, Tyberg JV. Pericardial pressure assessed by right atrial pressure: a basis for calculation of left ventricular transmural pressure. Am Heart J 1984;108:603–5.

25. Tyberg JV, Taichman GC, Smith ER, et al. The relationships between pericardial pressure and right atrial pressure: an intraoperative study. Circulation 1986;73:428–32.

26. Santamore WP, Constantinescu M, Little WC. Direct assessment of right ventricular transmural pressure. Circulation 1987;75:744–7.

27. Hamilton DR, Sas R, Semlacher RA, et al. The relationship between left and right pericardial pressures in humans: an intraoperative study. Can J Cardiol 2011;27(3):346–50.

28. Fewell JE, Abendschein DR, Carlson CJ, et al. Continuous positive pressure ventilation does not alter ventricular pressure-volume relationship. Am J Physiol 1981;240:H281–6.

29. Fewell JE, Abendschein DR, Carlson CJ, et al. Mechanism of decreased right and left ventricular end-diastolic volumes during continuous positive-pressure ventilation in dogs. Circ Res 1980;47: 467–72.

30. Tyberg JV. Mechanical modulation of cardiac function: role of the pericardium. In: Kohl P, Sachs F, Franz MR, editors. New Oxford textbook of cardiac mechano-electric feedback and arrhythmias. 2nd edition. Oxford, New York: Oxford University Press; 2011. p. 281–9.

31. Katz LN. Analysis of the several factors regulating the performance of the heart. Physiol Rev 1955; 35:91–106.

32. Molaug M, Stokland O, Ilebekk A, et al. Myocardial function of the interventricular septum. Effects of right and left ventricular pressure loading before and after pericardiotomy in dogs. Circ Res 1981;49:52–61.

33. Piene H, Myhre ES. Position of interventricular septum during heart cycle in anesthetized dogs. Am J Physiol 1991;260:H158–64.

34. Dell'Italia LJ, Pearce DJ, Blackwell GG, et al. Right and left ventricular volumes and function after acute pulmonary hypertension in the intact dog. J Appl Physiol 1995;78:2320–7.

35. Santamore WP, Dell'Italia LJ. Ventricular interdependence: significant left ventricular contributions to right ventricular systolic function. Prog Cardiovasc Dis 1998;40:289–308.

36. Laks MM, Garner D, Swan HJ. Volumes and compliances measured simultaneously in the right and left ventricles of the dog. Circ Res 1967;20: 565–9.

37. Taylor RR, Covell JW, Sonnenblick EH, et al. Dependence of ventricular distensibility on filling of the opposite ventricle. Am J Physiol 1967;213(3):711–8.

38. Bemis CE, Serur JR, Borkenhagen D, et al. Influence of right ventricular filling pressure on left ventricular pressure and dimension. Circ Res 1974;34(4):498–504.

39. Santamore WP, Lynch PR, Heckman JL, et al. Left ventricular effect on right ventricular developed pressure. J Appl Physiol 1976;41(6):925–30.

40. Spadaro J, Bing OH, Gaasch WH, et al. Pericardial modulation of right and left ventricular diastolic interaction. Circ Res 1981;48:233–8.

41. Janicki JS, Weber KT. The pericardium and ventricular interaction, distensibility, and function. Am J Physiol 1980;238:H494–503.

42. Maruyama Y, Ashikawa K, Isoyama S, et al. Mechanical interactions between four heart chambers with and without the pericardium in canine hearts. Circ Res 1982;50:86–100.

43. Glantz SA, Misbach GA, Moores WY, et al. The pericardium substantially affects the left ventricular diastolic pressure-volume relationship in the dog. Circ Res 1978;42(3):433–41.

44. Hess OM, Bhargava V, Ross J, et al. The role of the pericardium in interactions between the cardiac chambers. Am Heart J 1983;106:1377–83.

45. Lorell BH, Palacios I, Daggett WM, et al. Right ventricular distension and left ventricular compliance. Am J Physiol 1981;240:H87–98.

46. Tyberg JV, Misbach GA, Glantz SA, et al. A mechanism for shifts of the left ventricular pressure-volume curve: the role of the pericardium. Eur J Cardiol 1978;7S:163–75.

47. Shirato K, Shabetai R, Bhargava V, et al. Alteration of the left ventricular diastolic pressure-segment length relation produced by the pericardium, effects of cardiac distension and afterload reduction in conscious dogs. Circulation 1978;57(6):1191–8.

48. Tyson GS, Maier GW, Olsen CO, et al. Pericardial influences on ventricular filling in the conscious dog, an analysis based on pericardial pressure. Circ Res 1984;54:173–84.

49. Thames MD, Alpert JS, Dalen JE. Syncope in patients with pulmonary embolism. JAMA 1977; 238:2509–11.

50. Dexter L. Clinical aspects of pulmonary embolism and their relation to pathophysiology. Bull Physiopathol Respir 1970;6:21–34.

51. Miller GAH, Sutton GC. Acute massive pulmonary embolism: clinical and haemodynamic findings in 23 patients studied by cardiac catheterization and pulmonary arteriography. Br Heart J 1970;32:518–23.

52. Gardin F, Gurdjian F, Desfonds P, et al. Hemodynamic factors influencing arterial hypoxemia in massive pulmonary embolism with circulatory failure. Circulation 1979;59:909–12.

53. Visner MS, Arentzen CE, O'Connor MJ, et al. Alterations in left ventricular three-dimensional dynamic geometry and systolic function during acute right ventricular hypertension in the conscious dog. Circulation 1983;67(2):353–65.

54. Taquini AC, Fermoso JD, Aramendia P. Behavior of the right ventricle following acute constriction of the pulmonary artery. Circ Res 1960;8:315–8.

55. Badke FR. Left ventricular dimensions and function during right ventricular pressure overload. Am J Physiol 1982;242(4):H611–8.

56. Kingma I, Tyberg JV, Smith ER. Effects of diastolic transseptal pressure gradient on ventricular septal position and motion. Circulation 1983;69(6):1304–14.

57. Ghignone M, Girling L, Prewitt RM. Effect of increased pulmonary vascular resistance on right ventricular systolic performance in dogs. Am J Physiol 1984;246(3 Pt 2):H339–43.

58. Belenkie I, Dani R, Smith ER, et al. Ventricular interaction during experimental acute pulmonary embolism. Circulation 1988;78:761–8.

59. Belenkie I, Sas R, Mitchell J, et al. Opening the pericardium during pulmonary artery constriction improves cardiac function. J Appl Physiol 2004; 96:917–22.

60. Ludbrook PA, Byrne JD, Kurnik PB, et al. Influence of right ventricular hemodynamics on left ventricular diastolic pressure-volume relations in man. Circulation 1979;59:21–31.

61. Dell'Italia LJ, Walsh RA. Right ventricular diastolic pressure-volume relations and regional dimensions during acute alterations in loading conditions. Circulation 1988;77:1276–82.

62. Singh SF, White FC, Bloor CM. Myocardial morphometric characteristics in swine. Circ Res 1981;49: 434–41.

63. Marchetti G, Merlo L, Noseda V. Coronary sinus outflow and O_2 content in anterior cardiac vein blood at different levels of right ventricle performance. Pflugers Arch 1969;310:116–27.

64. Kusachi S, Nishiyama O, Yasuhara K, et al. Right and left ventricular oxygen metabolism in open-chest dogs. Am J Physiol 1982;243(5):H761–6.

65. Takeda K, Haraoka S, Nagashima H. Myocardial oxygen metabolism of the right ventricle with volume loading and hypoperfusion. Japanese Circ J 1987;51:563–72.

66. Saito D, Yamada N, Kusachi S, et al. Coronary flow reserve and oxygen metabolism of the right ventricle. Japanese Circ J 1989;53:1310–6.

67. Zong P, Tune JD, Downey HF. Mechanisms of oxygen demand/supply balance in the right ventricle. Exp Biol Med (Maywood) 2005;230(8):507–19.

68. Saito D, Tani H, Kusachi S, et al. Oxygen metabolism of the hypertrophic right ventricle in open chest dogs. Cardiovasc Res 1991;25(9):731–9.

69. Kolin A, Ross G, Gaal P, et al. Simultaneous electromagnetic measurement of blood flow in the major coronary arteries. Nature 1964;203(4941):148–50.

70. Ross G. Blood flow in the right coronary artery of the dog. Cardiovasc Res 1967;1:138–44.

71. Aukland K, Kiil F, Kjekshus J. Relationship between ventricular pressures and right and left myocardial blood flow. Acta Physiol Scand 1967;70:116–26.

72. Bellamy RF, Lowensohn HS. Effect of systole on coronary pressure-flow relations in the right ventricle of the dog. Am J Physiol 1980;238(4):H481–6.

73. Cross CE. Right ventricular pressure and coronary flow. Am J Physiol 1962;202(1):12–6.

74. Hess DS, Bache RJ. Transmural right ventricular myocardial blood flow during systole in the awake dog. Circ Res 1979;45(1):88–94.

75. Lowensohn HS, Khouri EM, Gregg DE, et al. Phasic right coronary artery blood flow in conscious dogs with normal and elevated right ventricular pressures. Circ Res 1976;39(6):760–6.

76. Peter RH, Ramo BW, Ratliff N, et al. Collateral vessel development after right ventricular infarction in the pig. Am J Cardiol 1972;29:56–60.

77. Meyer P, Filippatos GS, Ahmed MI, et al. Effects of right ventricular ejection fraction on outcomes in chronic systolic heart failure. Circulation 2010; 121:252–8.

78. Wang GY, McCloskey DT, Turcato S, et al. Contrasting inotropic responses to alpha1-adrenergic receptor stimulation in left versus right ventricular myocardium. Am J Physiol 2006;291:H2013–7.

79. Wang GY, Yeh CC, Hensen BC, et al. Heart failure switches the RV α1-adrenergic inotropic response from negative to positive. Am J Physiol 2010;298: H213–20.

80. Tanaka H, Manita S, Matsuda T, et al. Sustained negative inotropism mediated by alpha-adrenoceptors in adult mouse myocardia: developmental conversion from positive response in the neonate. Br J Pharmacol 1995;114:673–7.

81. Jensen BC, Swigart PM, De Marco T, et al. Alpha-1-adrenergic receptor subtypes in nonfailing and failing human myocardium. Circ Heart Fail 2009;2:654–63.

82. Milnor W, Bergel D, Bargainer J. Hydraulic power associated with pulmonary blood flow and its relation to heart rate. Circ Res 1966;19(3):467–80.

83. Milnor WR, Conti CR, Lewis KB, et al. Pulmonary arterial pulse wave velocity and impedance in man. Circ Res 1969;25(6):637–49.

84. O'Rourke MF. Vascular impedance in studies of arterial and cardiac function. Physiol Rev 1982; 62(2):570–623.

85. Piene H. Pulmonary arterial impedance and right ventricular function. Physiol Rev 1986;66(3):606–52.

86. van den Bos GC, Westerhof N, Randall OS. Pulse wave reflection: can it explain the differences between systemic and pulmonary pressure and flow waves? A study in dogs. Circ Res 1982;51: 479–85.

87. Bargainer JD. Pulse wave velocity in the main pulmonary artery of the dog. Circ Res 1967;20: 630–7.

88. Bergel DH, Milnor WR. Pulmonary vascular impedance in the dog. Circ Res 1965;16(5):401–15.

89. Murgo JP, Westerhof N. Input impedance of the pulmonary arterial system in normal man. Effects of respiration and comparison to systemic impedance. Circ Res 1984;54:666–73.

90. Caro CG, Harrison GK, Mognoni P. Pressure wave transmission in the human pulmonary circulation. Cardiovasc Res 1967;1:91–100.

91. Reuben SR. Wave transmission in the pulmonary arterial system in disease in man. Circ Res 1970; 27:523–9.

92. Elzinga G, Westerhof N. Pressure and flow generated by the left ventricle against different impedances. Circ Res 1973;32:178–86.

93. Elzinga G, Piene H, De Jong JP. Left and right ventricular pump function and consequences of having two pumps in one heart. Circ Res 1980; 46:564–74.

94. Dell'Italia LJ, Walsh RA. Acute determinants of the hangout interval in the pulmonary circulation. Am Heart J 1988;116:1289–97.

95. Dell'Italia LJ, Santamore WP. Can indices of left ventricular function be applied to the right ventricle? Prog Cardiovasc Dis 1998;40(4):309–24.

96. Dell'Italia LJ, Walsh RA. Application of a time varying elastance model to right ventricular performance in man. Cardiovasc Res 1988;22:864–74.

97. Mason DT. Usefulness and limitations of the rate of rise of intraventricular pressure (dP/dt) in the evaluation of myocardial contractility in man. Am J Cardiol 1969;23:516–27.

98. Wildenthal K, Mierzwiak DS, Mitchell JH. Effect of sudden changes in aortic pressure on left ventricular dP/dt. Am J Physiol 1969;216:185–90.

99. Gleason WL, Braunwald E. Studies on the first derivative of the ventricular pressure pulse in man. J Clin Invest 1962;41(1):80–91.

100. Stein PD, Sabbah HN, Anbe DT, et al. Performance of the failing and nonfailing right ventricle of patients with pulmonary hypertension. Am J Cardiol 1979;44:1050–5.

101. Piene H, Covell JW. Local auxotonic systolic force and work in canine right ventricular free wall. Am J Physiol 1983;244:H186–93.

102. Santamore WP, Meier GD, Bove AA. Effects of hemodynamic alterations on wall motion in the canine right ventricle. Am J Physiol 1979;236(2): H254–62.

103. Meier GD, Bove AA, Santamore WP, et al. Contractile function in canine right ventricle. Am J Physiol 1980;239:H794–804.

104. Raines RA, LeWinter MM, Covell JW. Regional shortening patterns in canine right ventricle. Am J Physiol 1976;231(5):1395–400.

105. Armour JA, Pace JB, Randall WC. Interrelationship of architecture and function of the right ventricle. Am J Physiol 1970;218(1):174–9.

106. Pace JB, Keefe WF, Armour JA, et al. Influence of sympathetic nerve stimulation on right ventricular outflow-tract pressures in anesthetized dogs. Circ Res 1969;24:397–407.

107. Pouleur H, Lefèvre J, Mechelen HV, et al. Free-wall shortening and relaxation during ejection in the canine right ventricle. Am J Physiol 1980;239:H601–13.

108. Noble IM. The contribution of blood momentum to left ventricular ejection in the dog. Circ Res 1968; 23:663–70.

109. Spencer MP, Griess FC. Dynamics of ventricular ejection. Circ Res 1962;10:274–9.

110. Raizada V, Sahn DJ, Covell JW. Factors influencing late right ventricular ejection. Cardiovasc Res 1988;22:244–8.

111. Oboler AA, Keefe JF, Gaasch WH, et al. Influence of left ventricular isovolumic pressure upon right ventricular isovolumic pressure and right ventricular pressure transients. Cardiology 1973;58:32–44.

112. Fenely MP, Gavaghan TP, Baron DW, et al. Contribution of left ventricular contraction to the generation of right ventricular systolic pressure in the human heart. Circulation 1985;71:473–80.

113. Langille BL, Jones DR. Mechanical interactions between the ventricles during systole. Can J Physiol Pharmacol 1977;55(3):373–82.

114. Rose JC, Cosimano SJ Jr, Hufnagel CA, et al. The effects of exclusion of the right ventricle from the circulation in dogs. J Clin Invest 1955; 34:1625–31.

115. Rose JC, Lazaro EJ, Broida HP. Dynamics of complete right ventricular failure in dogs maintained with an extracorporeal left ventricle. Circ Res 1956;4:173–81.

116. Puga FJ, McGoon DC. Exclusion of the right ventricle from the circulation: hemodynamic observations. Surgery 1973;73(4):607–13.

117. Furey SA III, Zieske HA, Levy MN. The essential function of the right ventricle. Am Heart J 1984; 107(2):404–10.

118. Sawatani S, Mandell C, Kusaba E. Ventricular performance following ablation and prosthetic replacement of right ventricular myocardium. Trans Am Artif Intern Organs 1974;20B:629–36.

119. Seki S, Ohba O, Tanizaki M, et al. Construction of a new right ventricle on the epicardium: a possible correction for underdevelopment of the right ventricle. J Thorac Cardiovasc Surg 1975;70(2):330–7.

120. Seki S, Ono K, Tanizaki M. Role of contraction and size of right ventricular free wall in performance of the heart. Jpn J Thorac Surg 1976;29(10):731–4.

121. Pennington DG, Merjavy JP, Swartz MT, et al. The importance of biventricular failure in patients with post operative cardiogenic shock. Ann Thorac Surg 1985;39:16–26.

122. Miyamoto AT, Tanaka S, Matloff JM. Right ventricular function during right heart bypass. J Thorac Cardiovasc Surg 1983;85:49–53.

123. Moulopoulos SD, Sarcas A, Stamatelopoulos S, et al. Left ventricular performance during bypass or distension of the right ventricle. Circ Res 1965; 17:484–91.

124. Suga H, Sawgawa K, Shoukas AA. Load independence of the instantaneous pressure-volume ratio of the canine left ventricle and effects of epinephrine and heart rate on the ratio. Circ Res 1973;32:314–22.

125. Suga H, Sagawa KP. Instantaneous pressure-volume relationships and their ratio in the excised, supported canine left ventricle. Circ Res 1974;35:117–26.

126. Maughan WL, Shoukas AA, Sagawa K, et al. Instantaneous pressure-volume relationship of the canine right ventricle. Circ Res 1979;44:309–15.

127. Brown KA, Ditchey RV. Human right ventricular end-systolic pressure-volume relation defined by maximal elastance. Circulation 1988;78:81–91.

128. Starling MR, Walsh RA, Dell'Italia LJ, et al. The relationship of various measures of end-systole to left ventricular maximum time-varying elastance in man. Circulation 1987;76(1):32–43.

129. Kono A, Maughan WL, Sunagawa K, et al. The use of left ventricular end-ejection pressure and peak pressure in the estimation of the end-systolic pressure-volume relationship. Circulation 1984;70:1057–65.

130. Pidgeon J, Miller GA, Noble MI, et al. The relationship between the strength of the human heart beat and the interval between beats. Circulation 1982; 65:1404–10.

131. Anderson PA, Manring A, Serwer GA, et al. The force-interval relationship of the left ventricle. Circulation 1979;60:334–48.

132. Wisenbaugh T, Nissen S, DeMaria A. Mechanics of postextrasystolic potentiation in normal subjects and patients with valvular heart disease. Circulation 1986;74:10–20.

133. Yue DT, Burkhoff D, Franz MR, et al. Postextrasystolic potentiation of the isolated canine left ventricle. Relationship to mechanical restitution. Circ Res 1985;56:340–50.

134. Burkhoff D, Yue DT, Franc MR, et al. Quantitative comparison of the force-interval relationships of the canine right and left ventricles. Circulation 1984;54: 468–73.

135. Dell'Italia LJ. Mechanism of postextrasystolic potentiation in the right ventricle. Am J Cardiol 1990;65:736–41.

Imaging of the Right Ventricle

Javier Sanz, MD[a],*, Jennifer Conroy, MD[b],
Jagat Narula, MD, PhD[a,b]

KEYWORDS

- Right ventricle • Imaging • Ultrasound • Nuclear medicine
- Computed tomography • Magnetic resonance

Focus on the roles of the right ventricle (RV) in cardiovascular homeostasis both in normal and pathologic conditions has lagged behind that of the left ventricle (LV) for a long time. In part, this has been because of the difficulties associated with imaging the RV in a noninvasive fashion, particularly with echocardiography (**Box 1**). The significant impact of RV performance on patients' clinical status and outcome has been progressively realized over the past decades, however, leading to increased efforts in developing techniques that can reliably evaluate this chamber. The advent of 2-dimensional (2D) echocardiography clearly represented an important leap forward, allowing for the routine assessment of RV size and function in the clinical setting. Simultaneously, nuclear techniques provided a means for noninvasive measurement of these parameters in a more quantitative way. Two additional imaging modalities, computed tomography (CT) and, particularly, cardiac magnetic resonance (CMR), have more recently joined our armamentarium for RV evaluation. Unfortunately, there is no single technique to date that fulfills all characteristics that would constitute the ideal imaging modality (**Box 2**), and each has its own challenges, strengths, and limitations (**Table 1**). In this review, we discuss state-of-the-art imaging of the RV. Key points are summarized in **Box 3**.

CHEST RADIOGRAPHY

Still today, chest x-ray is often the first imaging test that the patient with suspected RV disease undergoes because of its low cost and wide availability. The lateral view is best suited for the detection of RV enlargement, which can be noted when the cardiac silhouette occupies more than 40% of the lower retrosternal space (**Fig. 1**A). RV enlargement also leads to posterior cardiac rotation and lateral displacement of the RV outflow tract, so that the pulmonary artery contour on the left cardiac border appears more prominent (see **Fig. 1**B). In addition, a simple chest x-ray can suggest concomitant abnormalities, such as right atrial dilatation, left heart disease, pulmonary congestion, or pulmonary parenchymal disease. Nonetheless, chest x-ray remains a very preliminary imaging tool for RV assessment that offers reasonable sensitivity but poor specificity.[1]

ECHOCARDIOGRAPHY

In clinical practice, ultrasound is by far the most common modality used to image the RV, and its use is generally considered appropriate for this application, particularly in the settings of pulmonary hypertension or acute coronary syndromes.[2] Echocardiography is portable, inexpensive, and

The authors have no disclosures to report.
[a] Zena and Michael A. Wiener Cardiovascular Institute and Marie-Josee and Henry R. Kravis Center for Cardiovascular Health, Mount Sinai School of Medicine, Box 1030, New York, NY 10029, USA; [b] Zena and Michael A. Wiener Cardiovascular Institute and Marie-Josee and Henry R. Kravis Center for Cardiovascular Health, Mount Sinai Hospital, One Gustave L Levy Place, Box 1030, New York, NY 10029, USA
* Corresponding author.
E-mail address: Javier.Sanz@mssm.edu

Box 1
Difficulties in RV imaging

- Complex shape, which limits the application of geometric models for volume-function quantification.
- Retrosternal position, which creates an acoustic barrier for ultrasound waves.
- Distinct embryologic origin and hemodynamic environment (high-volume, low-pressure system) that significantly differs from the LV and is associated with thinner walls and prominent trabeculations, which are more difficult to characterize.

---

widely available. Importantly, transthoracic echocardiography is, with the exception of the use of contrast, entirely noninvasive and poses little to no risk for the patient. Moreover, echocardiography has the ability to simultaneously assess biventricular and valvular function and provide important hemodynamic information from Doppler flow measurements. Limitations of echocardiography are related to the location, anatomy, and contractile mechanism of the RV, as summarized in **Box 1** and **Table 1**. In addition, many indices of RV performance are markedly load dependent.

There are many different echocardiographic techniques that can be combined for a comprehensive evaluation of the RV, as detailed in **Table 2**.

RV Size and Morphology

RV hypertrophy and dilatation

The accurate evaluation of RV size, volume, and contractility requires a complete set of standardized 2D images.[3] Pathologic changes reflecting RV pressure overload include hypertrophy and abnormal septal motion. A value of end-diastolic free wall thickness greater than 5 mm indicates hypertrophy, and is strongly associated with chronically increased afterload.[4] Over time, in the setting of pressure overload, RV contractile dysfunction and dilatation may develop. RV volumes are generally difficult to quantify because of the complex structure of the RV. Hence, 2D methods that rely on Simpson's formula suffer from lack of standardization and the tendency to underestimate volumes. Instead, visual estimation of the RV size relative to the LV or measurements of transverse and longitudinal lengths are often used (**Table 3**). In general, an RV diastolic area that approximates or exceeds that of the LV in the 4-chamber view suggests RV dilatation (**Fig. 2**).[5]

Interventricular septal configuration

In the setting of RV pressure overload, the interventricular septum becomes flattened and bows

---

Box 2
Characteristics of an ideal imaging modality

- High spatial and temporal resolution, to provide accurate measurement of dynamic changes in RV shape and size.
- High contrast-to-noise ratios, so that the RV can be easily differentiated from surrounding structures.
- Versatility, so that different anatomic and physiologic aspects of the RV can be evaluated, including tissue characterization and blood flow patterns.
- Ability to simultaneously provide information on other structures intimately related to RV performance, such as the left heart side and the pulmonary circulation.
- Complete noninvasiveness, including need for intravenous access.
- Harmlessness, including absence of potentially toxic contrast agents and ionizing radiation.
- Rapid acquisition, which may be particularly important for the sickest patients.
- Low cost of both performance and maintenance.
- Portability, so that the test can be performed at the bedside if needed.
- Widespread availability in both inpatient and outpatient settings.
- Accuracy, being validated to provide reliable quantification of measured indices.
- Reproducibility among readers and tests.
- Robustness, allowing for the reliable performance of the technique in a wide range of individuals and clinical scenarios.

Table 1
Relative strengths and limitations of different modalities for right ventricular imaging

	TTE	Nuclear	CT	CMR
Spatial resolution	++++	+	+++	++
Temporal resolution	++++	++	+	+++
Contrast resolution	+	++	+++	++++
Large field of view	+	+++	++++	++++
3D imaging	++	+	++++	+++
Accuracy	++	+	+++	++++
Versatility	+++	++	+	++++
Safety	++++	++	+	+++
Cost	++++	++	+++	+
Portability	++++	+	+	+
Robustness	++	+	+++	+++
Speed	+++	+	++++	++
Availability	++++	+++	++	+

A higher number of + signs indicates better performance.
Abbreviations: CMR, cardiac magnetic resonance; CT, computed tomography; TTE, transthoracic echocardiography; 3D, 3-dimensional.

toward the LV, particularly during end-systole, with greater degrees of shift signifying more significant pressure overload. RV volume overload and enlargement may also produce flattening and shifting of the interventricular septum, which is seen primarily in diastole and is most marked at the end of it. Septal bowing toward the left leads to LV underfilling and reduced stroke volume, even in the presence of normal systolic function. The LV eccentricity index is calculated as the ratio of the anteroposterior to the septal-lateral short axis cavity dimension of the LV at either end-diastole or end-systole. Values greater than 1 reflect RV overload.[5,6] In addition, the degree of septal curvature and its relation to the LV free wall curvature can be used to estimate transeptal pressure gradients and RV systolic pressures.[7]

RV Hemodynamics

Although beyond the scope of this article, important information on right heart hemodynamics can be derived from echocardiographic images and are reviewed in detail elsewhere.[5] Quantification of RV systolic pressures is typically performed using the tricuspid regurgitant jet and the modified Bernoulli equation (**Fig. 3**). Alternative approaches include Doppler imaging of the RV outflow tract. In

---

Box 3
Key points

- Echocardiography remains the mainstay of RV imaging in clinical practice with methods such as fractional area shortening, tricuspid annular plane systolic motion, the Tei index, Doppler tissue imaging of the tricuspid annulus, or speckle tracking of the RV free wall.

- Emerging echocardiographic techniques include 3-dimensional ultrasound, which offers potential advantages for absolute quantification of RV volumes.

- CMR is the reference standard for the measurement of RV volumes and ejection fraction and also provides information regarding tissue characterization that has diagnostic and prognostic implications.

- Gated computed tomography is an excellent alternative method for quantitative RV assessment when echocardiography or CMR is inadequate or contraindicated.

- Nuclear techniques do not currently have a predominant role in RV evaluation, although data are emerging on the use of positron emission tomography for RV myocardial imaging.

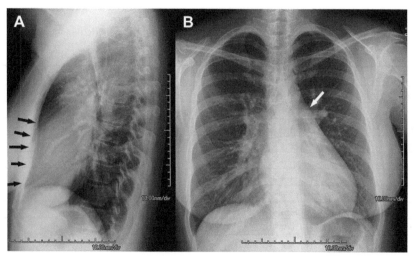

Fig. 1. (A) Lateral chest x-ray in a woman with large RV enlargement owing to severe systemic-to-pulmonary shunting. The dilated RV is indicated by the black arrows. (B) Posteroanterior chest x-ray demonstrated a prominent pulmonary artery contour (*white arrow*).

addition, right atrial pressure can be estimated from the inferior cava vein diameter and its response to respiratory changes.

RV Systolic Function

There are multiple approaches for measuring RV systolic function, as listed in **Table 4**. Emerging techniques include measures of RV strain and strain rates, speckle tracking, and the use of 3D echocardiography. In practice, however, a semi-quantitative approach based on visual assessment

is commonly used. Echocardiography may also provide evidence of specific underlying etiologies of RV dysfunction, such as arrhythmogenic RV dysplasia. Pathologic findings include global RV dysfunction, segmental wall motion abnormalities, localized free wall aneurysms, global RV dilatation, isolated RV outflow tract dilatation, and possibly increased tissue echogenicity.[8] More recently, the imaging criteria for the diagnosis of this disease have been updated into more quantitative and less operator-dependent indices, as detailed in **Table 5**.

Table 2
Echocardiographic methods for the assessment of the right ventricle

Method	Application
M-mode	RV wall thickness RV outflow tract shortening TAPSE
2D echo	Linear dimensions Visual assessment of volumes/ejection fraction Ventricular eccentricity index Fractional area change
Conventional Doppler	RV systolic pressures Myocardial performance index
Doppler tissue imaging	Myocardial performance index IVA Strain and strain rate
Speckle tracking	Strain and strain rate
3D echo	RV volumes RV Ejection Fraction

Abbreviations: D, dimensional; IVA, isovolumic acceleration; RV, right ventricle; TAPSE, tricuspid annular plane systolic excursion.

Table 3 Normal RV echocardiographic dimensions in adults[a]	
Dimension	Normal Range, cm
RV length (base-to-apex)	7.1–7.9
Basal RV	2.0–2.8
Mid RV	2.7–3.3
RV outflow tract	2.5–2.9
Pulmonary artery	1.5–2.1

Abbreviation: RV, right ventricle.
  [a] Reference values taken from Mertens and Friedberg.[6]

RV fractional area change
The fractional area change is the percentage of change in the RV chamber area in an apical 4-chamber view during the cardiac cycle, and seems to be the 2D parameter that correlates best with CMR.[9] The RV fractional area change is an independent predictor of adverse events following myocardial infarction.[10,11]

Tricuspid annular plane systolic excursion
Tricuspid annular plane systolic excursion (TAPSE) is an assessment of longitudinal RV function measured with the M-mode in the apical 4-chamber view. A value of less than 1.6 cm indicates RV dysfunction and has been proven to predict mortality in pulmonary hypertension.[5,12] This method shows a strong correlation with radionuclide angiography RV ejection fraction, although it correlated poorly with CMR.[9,13] Although fast and simple, it is a 1D approach, reflecting only regional (basal) RV systolic function. Despite these limitations, recent guidelines from the American Society of Echocardiography recommend that "TAPSE should be used routinely" in the assessment of RV function.[5]

RV index of myocardial performance
The RV index of myocardial performance (RIMP), or Tei index, is a measure of global RV systolic and diastolic function. It is calculated as the ratio of the total RV isovolumic time divided by the RV ejection time.[14] The normal value is 0.28 ± 0.04. Values greater than 0.40 by pulsed wave Doppler and greater than 0.55 by tissue Doppler reflect RV dysfunction.[5] The RIMP has shown significant correlation with RV ejection fraction by nuclear ventriculography and is also less affected by loading conditions and heart rate.[14,15]

Doppler tissue imaging
Pulsed Doppler tissue imaging (DTI) quantifies peak velocities. The tricuspid lateral annular systolic velocity (S′) is obtained with the use of pulsed DTI at the tricuspid annulus (**Fig. 4**). A value of S′ below 9.7 cm/s suggests abnormal RV contractility,[16] and may be useful in the detection of early RV dysfunction.[17] S′ is also lower in patients with idiopathic pulmonary hypertension than in healthy controls, and is inversely related to pulmonary pressures and resistance.[18] In addition, there are good correlations between DTI of the tricuspid annulus and RV ejection fraction quantified by radionuclide angiography.[19]

Color DTI acquires color-coded images of the RV, which represent average velocities within a specific region of interest. Color DTI may also be used to obtain S′, although it is primarily a research tool and with less validation for clinical application. Recent advances in the echocardiographic evaluation of RV function include assessment of RV strain and strain rate. Strain is a measure of tissue deformation, whereas strain rate is a measure of deformation over time.[20] Strain measures can be also obtained with the use of DTI. Strain imaging has been limited to the apical 4-chamber view (longitudinal strain), whereas circumferential strain is assessed in short axis view and remains investigational. Compared with spectral DTI, color DTI improves spatial resolution of RV wall motion; however, it still remains largely a research tool because of angle and frame rate dependence, complex postprocessing, low temporal resolution, and relative lack of experience.

Isovolumic acceleration, or myocardial acceleration during isovolumetric contraction, is a newer parameter of global RV systolic function, calculated as the maximal isovolumetric myocardial velocity divided by time to peak velocity.[5,21] Although it appears to be less load dependent than other methods,[22] its routine use in the

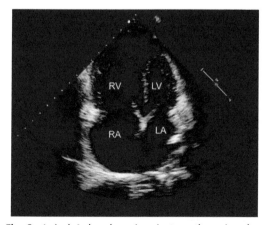

Fig. 2. Apical 4-chamber view in transthoracic echocardiogram demonstrating marked RV dilatation. LA, left atrium; LV, left ventricle; RA, right atrium; RV, right ventricle.

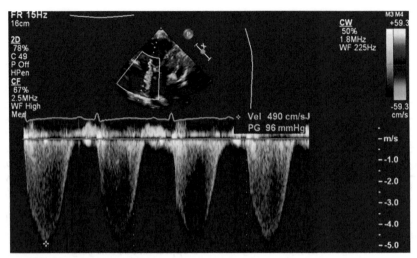

Fig. 3. Continuous wave Doppler recording of the tricuspid regurgitant jet demonstrating a peak velocity (crosshair) of 4.9 m/s or, by using the modified Bernoulli equation, the peak gradient (PG) = $4V^2$ or 96 mm Hg. With an estimated right atrial pressure of 10 mm Hg, the RV systolic pressure is 106 mm Hg.

assessment of RV systolic function is not recommended, as there are limited data and no standard reference ranges.[5]

Speckle tracking
Speckle tracking analyzes motion by tracking speckles in the myocardium with an algorithm that identifies speckle location on sequential frames (velocity vector imaging) and derives strain values (**Fig. 5**). It is less dependent on 2D image quality, frame rate and angle, and has the ability to measure RV strain in both long and short axis planes. Several studies have shown that it is a feasible and accurate method to assess global and regional RV function in healthy volunteers and patients with pulmonary hypertension.[23,24]

Table 4
Indices of RV systolic function in adults

Method	Abnormal[a]	Limitations
2D RV EF	<44%	Multiple methods; unreliable
FAC	<35%	Requires accurate tracing of endocardial border
TAPSE	<1.6 cm	Angle dependent Load dependent
RIMP		Unreliable with irregular heart rates or elevated RA pressures
Pulsed	>0.44	
Tissue	>0.55	
IVA	No recommended reference	Limited data Angle dependent Varies with heart rate and age Load dependent
S' (pulsed)	<10 cm/s	Angle dependent Assumes all segments have similar function Limited data for use in elderly
3D EF	<44%	Time consuming Less commonly available

Abbreviations: EF, ejection fraction; FAC, fractional area change; IVA, isovolumic acceleration; RA, right atrium; RIMP, RV index of myocardial performance; RV, right ventricle; S', tricuspid lateral annular systolic velocity; TAPSE, tricuspid annular plane systolic excursion.
  [a] Reference values taken from American Society of Echocardiography.[5]

Table 5
Revised imaging criteria for diagnosis of arrhythmogenic cardiomyopathy

	Major Criteria	Minor Criteria
TTE	Regional RV akinesis, dyskinesis or aneurysm *plus* one of: • RVOT ≥19 mm/m² (PLAX) • RVOT ≥21 mm/m² (PSAX) • FAC ≤33%	Regional RV akinesis or dyskinesis *plus* one of: • RVOT = 16–18 mm/m² (PLAX) • RVOT = 18–20 mm/m² (PSAX) • FAC = 34%–40%
CMR	Regional RV akinesis, dyskinesis or RV dyssynchronny *plus* one of: • RVEDV ≥110 mL/m² (male) or ≥100 mL/m² (female) • RVEF ≤40%	Regional RV akinesis, dyskinesis or RV dyssynchronny *plus* one of: • RVEDV = 100–109 mL/m² (male) or 90–99 mL/m² (female) • RVEF 41%–45%
RV angiography	Regional RV akinesis, dyskinesis or aneurysm	

Abbreviations: CMR, cardiac magnetic resonance; FAC, fractional area change; PLAX, parasternal long axis; PSAX, parasternal short axis; RV, right ventricle; RVEDV, right ventricular end-diastolic volume; RVEF, right ventricular ejection fraction; RVOT, right ventricular outflow tract.

Data from Marcus FI, McKenna WJ, Sherrill D, et al. Diagnosis of arrhythmogenic right ventricular cardiomyopathy/dysplasia: proposed modification of the task force criteria. Circulation 2010;121:1533–41.

Diastolic Function

Regarding RV diastolic function, in addition to assessing right atrial size, myocardial DTI in combination with pulsed wave Doppler analysis of the tricuspid inflow may be a useful modality, allowing the quantification of the E/A, E/E′, and E′/A′ ratios. Another method relies on measuring the isovolumic relaxation time, which is prolonged in the setting of diastolic dysfunction.[5,6,21,25]

Three-Dimensional Echocardiography

The introduction of new matrix transducers, as well as advances in image acquisition and analysis have increased the use of real-time 3D echocardiography in the clinical setting. There are still limitations related to limited temporal resolution of real-time imaging or the need to average 4 to 7 cardiac cycles with full-volume imaging, which may cause artifacts in cases of arrhythmia. Direct visualization of

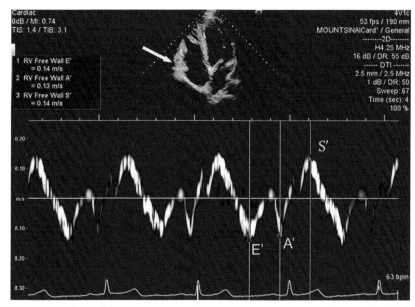

Fig. 4. Doppler tissue imaging of the lateral tricuspid annulus (*arrow*). Myocardial systolic (S′) and diastolic (E′ and A′) velocities can be obtained.

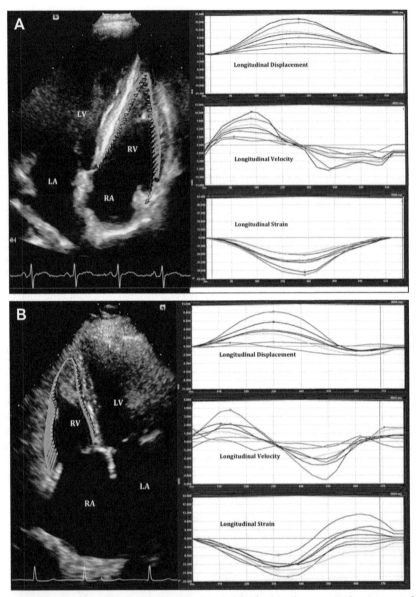

Fig. 5. Velocity vector imaging showing (*A*) normal and (*B*) abnormal segmental patterns of longitudinal displacement, velocity, and strain. LA, left atrium; LV, left ventricle; RA, right atrium; RV, right ventricle. (*Courtesy of* Dr Partho Sengupta and Dr Giuseppe Caracciolo.)

the entire RV with 3D echocardiography is possible using the full-volume mode acquisition. This capability is particularly attractive for the RV, as it has the potential advantage to measure cardiac chambers without geometric assumptions. Both older[26] and more recent real-time 3D techniques[27,28] have been validated for RV volume quantification, and may provide important mechanistic and prognostic value in various clinical scenarios, such as congenital heart disease[29] or functional tricuspid regurgitation.[30] In addition, multiplane reconstruction analysis allows accurate evaluation of segmental RV geometry and function.

NUCLEAR IMAGING
RV Volumes and Function

First-pass radionuclide ventriculography relies on the detection of the transit of a [99m]Technetium-labeled tracer through the RV. A quality bolus injection that results in enough RV counts is crucial, and normal values have been reported as 52% ± 6% with a lower limit of normal of 40%.[31] Although it provides only 1 imaging plane, it is considered the nuclear method of choice for RV assessment because of reasonably good correlations with CMR.[32] Alternatively, RV function evaluation can be performed with gated equilibrium blood pool imaging over longer acquisition periods, which is technically less demanding. Planar imaging is limited because of overlap between the RV and adjacent chambers.[33] A promising although less validated alternative is tomographic imaging that provides a true 3D dataset and allows for better separation of cardiac chambers.[33] Nuclear techniques for RV volumes and function are nonetheless restricted by limited spatial resolution, relatively prolonged imaging times, and need for radioisotopes. Thus, they are not routinely used for RV imaging in most centers and their use is not currently considered appropriate.[34]

Myocardial Characterization

Similarly, the small thickness of the normal RV wall limits the application of nuclear techniques for RV myocardial characterization; however, positron emission tomography (PET) has been successfully used recently to characterize RV myocardial metabolism with ^{18}F-fluorodeoxyglucose (FDG) in patients with left heart failure. The RV-to-LV ratio of FDG uptake is negatively correlated to RV ejection fraction.[35] Imaging is easier to perform in the presence of RV hypertrophy, such as that seen in pulmonary hypertension. This has enabled the detection of inducible RV ischemia with single-photon emission computed tomography in patients with idiopathic pulmonary hypertension.[36] In addition, studies using PET have demonstrated correlations between RV FDG accumulation and the degrees of pulmonary hypertension severity and RV overload, and potential for serial imaging of the effects of therapy.[37,38] It is possible that this increase in FDG uptake signals a metabolic shift from fatty acid to glucose use as a source of energy, a compensatory but maladaptive mechanism in early stages of ventricular failure. Increased FDG uptake also may be seen in inflammatory disorders, such as myocarditis or sarcoidosis (**Fig. 6**).[39] Less commonly, gallium-67

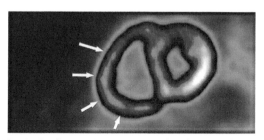

Fig. 6. Cardiac PET in a patient with pulmonary hypertension and sarcoidosis. Note the increased uptake in the thickened RV free wall (*white arrows*) as well as focal areas of increased uptake. (*Courtesy of* Dr Joseph Machac.)

scintigraphy may be used to detect inflammation with high specificity but low sensitivity.[40]

INVASIVE ANGIOGRAPHY

RV cineangiograms can be acquired during the injection of iodinated contrast through a pigtail or similar catheter positioned in the RV cavity. Typically, 2 separate orthogonal views are acquired (**Fig. 7**). With these views, RV volumes and function can be quantified using Simpson's rule[41] or simplified analytical approaches[42] that still require geometric assumptions. In addition, it can be combined with concomitant assessment of pulmonary hemodynamics or pulmonary angiography. Because of its invasive nature, cost, and associated risk, contrast ventriculography is rarely used in routine clinical practice with the possible exception of the patient with congenital heart disease in the setting of planned percutaneous interventions. Ventriculography-related complications, such as arrhythmias or acute volume overload, are more common in the presence of severe RV dysfunction and are associated with morbidity and mortality rates of 3.5% and 0.5%, respectively.[43]

COMPUTED TOMOGRAPHY
Non-gated CT

Beyond its widespread use for the evaluation of pulmonary vascular disease, contrast-enhanced CT can provide valuable information regarding RV status. In the setting of an acute pulmonary embolism, a right-left maximal ventricular diameter ratio greater than 0.9 in a reformatted 4-chamber view is an independent predictor of 30-day mortality.[44] More recently, dilatation of the RV by 3D volume quantification has been identified as a stronger and independent predictor of early death in this setting. Furthermore, other markers of RV failure that portend poor outcome included interventricular septal displacement and the presence of contrast reflux in the inferior vena cava.[45]

Gated CT

Helical CT of the heart with retrospective electrocardiographic gating is accurate for the quantification of RV volumes and function when compared with CMR.[46] This requires performing short-axis reformations and tracing endocardial contours in a manner comparable with CMR, or the use of attenuation-based 3D methods. Although the feasibility of evaluating RV dysfunction in patients with an acute pulmonary embolism or pulmonary hypertension has been reported,[47] its prognostic significance has not

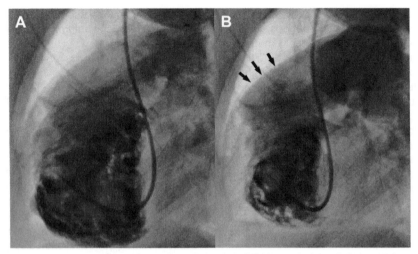

Fig. 7. Lateral RV contrast ventriculography in diastole (*panel A*) and systole (*panel B*) in an infant with repaired tetralogy of Fallot. There is an akinetic area in the RV outflow tract corresponding to the surgical patch (*arrows*).

been tested systematically. Because of the need for potentially nephrotoxic contrast agents and ionizing radiation, CT is rarely used solely for RV function evaluation; however, it is currently considerate an appropriate indication.[48] CT is particularly useful when echocardiography and CMR are inadequate or contraindicated. This includes patients with heart failure carrying an LV assist device, where RV performance is an important determinant of outcome and where CT quantification of RV function and volumes is feasible and reproducible.[49] An additional situation where CT can provide valuable information is in the adult patient with complex congenital heart disease in the presence of pacemakers or defibrillators (**Fig. 8**).[50] Beyond quantification of volumes or function, evolving applications of CT include evaluation of segmental wall abnormalities and/or fatty infiltration in arrhythmogenic RV dysplasia.[51] It must be noted, however, that the presence of fat in the RV wall can be seen in healthy individuals.[52]

MAGNETIC RESONANCE
General RV Evaluation

In the past decade, advances in CMR have significantly improved our ability to image the RV. The combination of high-resolution, unlimited imaging planes and absence of "acoustic" window limitations results in robust and accurate measurements of RV volumes and ejection fraction, for which CMR is currently considered the reference standard,[17] and its use regarded as appropriate.[53] Cine imaging is typically performed in contiguous short-axis views from base to apex, allowing for quantification using Simpson's method and

without geometric assumptions. Because function evaluation does not require contrast and has high reproducibility and excellent safety, CMR is well suited for serial evaluations.[54] More sophisticated analyses of RV performance can be obtained in specialized centers deriving RV volume/pressure loops by concomitant use of CMR-compatible catheters.[55] Additional applications include visual or quantitative evaluation of segmental function, tissue characterization with depiction of fatty infiltration or, after contrast administration, of myocardial scarring (**Table 6**). The main limitations of CMR are higher cost, reduced availability and

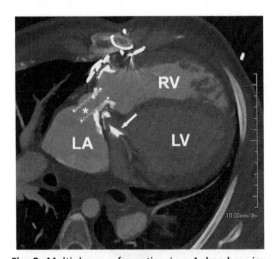

Fig. 8. Multiplanar reformation in a 4-chamber view orientation of cardiac CT in a patient with transposition of the great arteries status post Mustard repair, demonstrating RV hypertrophy. The left atrium (LA) connects to the systemic ventricle (the RV) through a narrowed baffle with a patent stent (*asterisk*). A pacemaker lead (*arrow*) is noted entering the LV.

Table 6
CMR sequences and applications in RV evaluation

Sequence	Application
Cine imaging	RV volumes, mass, and ejection fraction
Tagging Myocardial phase-contrast imaging Strain-encoded imaging	Segmental RV function[a]
Pulmonary artery phase-contrast imaging	Pulmonary flow/stiffness
T1-weighted spin-echo imaging	Myocardial fatty infiltration
Delayed postcontrast enhancement	Myocardial scarring

Abbreviations: CMR, cardiac magnetic resonance; RV, right ventricle.
  [a] Typically used only in research studies.

expertise, and safety constraints related to the magnetic field.

Specific Scenarios

Pulmonary hypertension

CMR is increasingly used to quantify the severity of RV enlargement, hypertrophy, and systolic dysfunction in pulmonary hypertension (**Fig. 9**). An RV-to-LV mass ratio greater than 0.6 was 84% sensitive and 71% specific for the diagnosis.[56] Moreover, an RV end-diastolic volume index greater than or equal to 84 mL/m^2 and LV end-diastolic volume index less than or equal to 40 mL/m^2 have been identified as predictors of 1-year mortality in idiopathic pulmonary hypertension.[57] Systolic dysfunction appears to develop earlier and more severely in the apex,

a finding that could have implications for early detection.[58] The combination of cine imaging of the RV with flow information from the pulmonary artery allows for the evaluation of the influence of arterial stiffness on RV performance,[59] improved detection of pulmonary hypertension,[60] and quantification of hemodynamic indices of load and ventriculoarterial coupling.[61,62] In addition, interventricular septal curvature can be quantified and leftward septal bowing has been associated with a systolic pulmonary artery pressure higher than 67 mm Hg.[63] Furthermore, the ratio of septal to LV free wall curvatures allows for noninvasive quantification of systolic pulmonary artery pressure.[64] Finally, focal of fibrosis is often present in the septum at the RV insertion points, a finding that correlates with pulmonary hypertension severity[65] but is of unclear (if any) clinical significance.

Arrhythmogenic cardiomyopathy

The evaluation of arrhythmogenic cardiomyopathy with CMR is considered an appropriate indication[53] and relies on the presence of RV enlargement and dysfunction together with characterization of the myocardium for the presence of fatty deposits or fibrosis. Although considerable emphasis has been placed on the detection of fatty infiltration, this finding has limited specificity and inter-reader agreement.[66] Visualization of fibrosis with delayed enhancement is feasible[67] but difficult, because of the small thickness of the RV free wall. Therefore, current diagnostic criteria are largely based on the presence of global or segmental dilatation or wall motion abnormalities (see **Table 5**).[68]

Congenital heart disease

CMR is optimally suited for RV evaluation in this setting, particularly in complex disease in adults, such as those with transposition of the great arteries or tetralogy of Fallot[69] in whom TTE may be substantially limited. In patients with repaired

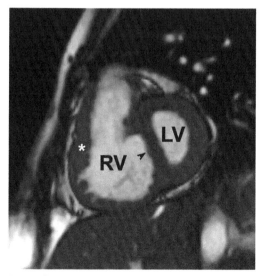

Fig. 9. Short axis CMR cine view in a patient with severe pulmonary hypertension. The right ventricle (RV) is severely dilated and hypertrophic (*asterisk*). There is septal flattening (*arrowhead*), resulting in D-shaped configuration of the LV.

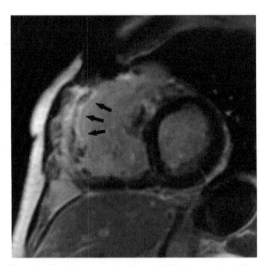

Fig. 10. Short-axis postcontrast CMR view in a patient with repaired tetralogy of Fallot. The RV is severely enlarged, and there is marked delayed enhancement (scarring) in the RV free wall (*arrows*).

tetralogy, RV cine and pulmonary artery flow imaging can be used to accurately quantify the degree of RV dilatation and of pulmonary regurgitation. An RV end-diastolic volume greater than 160 mL/m^2 or an end-systolic volume greater than 82 mL/m^2 have been associated with incomplete RV remodeling after pulmonary valve replacement.[70] In addition, the presence of myocardial scarring after tetralogy repair heralds an increased risk of adverse outcomes, including ventricular arrhythmias (**Fig. 10**).[71]

SUMMARY

Several imaging modalities can be used alone or in combination for a comprehensive evaluation of the RV. Echocardiography remains the mainstay modality because of its versatility, low cost, and widespread availability. CMR is the reference test for quantification of RV volumes and ejection fraction, and is also well suited for myocardial characterization. In patients in whom ultrasound and CMR are inadequate or contraindicated, CT represents a robust alternative for RV evaluation at the expense of contrast and radiation administration. The role of nuclear techniques on RV imaging is today limited, but there are emerging data on RV wall characterization with PET.

REFERENCES

1. Boxt LM. Radiology of the right ventricle. Radiol Clin North Am 1999;37:379–400.
2. Douglas PS, Khandheria B, Stainback RF, et al. ACCF/ ASE/ACEP/ASNC/SCAI/SCCT/SCMR 2007 appropriateness criteria for transthoracic and transesophageal echocardiography: a report of the American College of Cardiology Foundation Quality Strategic Directions Committee Appropriateness Criteria Working Group, American Society of Echocardiography, American College of Emergency Physicians, American Society of Nuclear Cardiology, Society for Cardiovascular Angiography and Interventions, Society of Cardiovascular Computed Tomography, and the Society for Cardiovascular Magnetic Resonance endorsed by the American College of Chest Physicians and the Society of Critical Care Medicine. J Am Coll Cardiol 2007;50:187–204.
3. Lang RM, Bierig M, Devereux RB, et al. Recommendations for chamber quantification: a report from the American Society of Echocardiography's Guidelines and Standards Committee and the Chamber Quantification Writing Group, developed in conjunction with the European Association of Echocardiography, a branch of the European Society of Cardiology. J Am Soc Echocardiogr 2005;18:1440–63.
4. Matsukubo H, Matsuura T, Endo N, et al. Echocardiographic measurement of right ventricular wall thickness. A new application of subxiphoid echocardiography. Circulation 1977;56:278–84.
5. Rudski LG, Lai WW, Afilalo J, et al. Guidelines for the echocardiographic assessment of the right heart in adults: a report from the American Society of Echocardiography endorsed by the European Association of Echocardiography, a registered branch of the European Society of Cardiology, and the Canadian Society of Echocardiography. J Am Soc Echocardiogr 2010;23:685–713 [quiz: 86–8].
6. Mertens LL, Friedberg MK. Imaging the right ventricle—current state of the art. Nat Rev Cardiol 2010;7:551–63.
7. King ME, Braun H, Goldblatt A, et al. Interventricular septal configuration as a predictor of right ventricular systolic hypertension in children: a cross-sectional echocardiographic study. Circulation 1983; 68:68–75.
8. Lindstrom L, Wilkenshoff UM, Larsson H, et al. Echocardiographic assessment of arrhythmogenic right ventricular cardiomyopathy. Heart 2001;86:31–8.
9. Anavekar NS, Gerson D, Skali H, et al. Two-dimensional assessment of right ventricular function: an echocardiographic-MRI correlative study. Echocardiography 2007;24:452–6.
10. Anavekar NS, Skali H, Bourgoun M, et al. Usefulness of right ventricular fractional area change to predict death, heart failure, and stroke following myocardial infarction (from the VALIANT ECHO Study). Am J Cardiol 2008;101:607–12.
11. Zornoff LA, Skali H, Pfeffer MA, et al. Right ventricular dysfunction and risk of heart failure and mortality after myocardial infarction. J Am Coll Cardiol 2002;39:1450–5.

12. Forfia PR, Fisher MR, Mathai SC, et al. Tricuspid annular displacement predicts survival in pulmonary hypertension. Am J Respir Crit Care Med 2006;174: 1034–41.

13. Ueti OM, Camargo EE, Ueti Ade A, et al. Assessment of right ventricular function with Doppler echocardiographic indices derived from tricuspid annular motion: comparison with radionuclide angiography. Heart 2002;88:244–8.

14. Tei C, Dujardin KS, Hodge DO, et al. Doppler echocardiographic index for assessment of global right ventricular function. J Am Soc Echocardiogr 1996; 9:838–47.

15. Karnati PK, El-Hajjar M, Torosoff M, et al. Myocardial performance index correlates with right ventricular ejection fraction measured by nuclear ventriculography. Echocardiography 2008;25:381–5.

16. Lindqvist P, Waldenstrom A, Henein M, et al. Regional and global right ventricular function in healthy individuals aged 20–90 years: a pulsed Doppler tissue imaging study: Umea General Population Heart Study. Echocardiography 2005;22:305–14.

17. Champion HC, Michelakis ED, Hassoun PM. Comprehensive invasive and noninvasive approach to the right ventricle-pulmonary circulation unit: state of the art and clinical and research implications. Circulation 2009;120:992–1007.

18. Ruan Q, Nagueh SF. Clinical application of tissue Doppler imaging in patients with idiopathic pulmonary hypertension. Chest 2007;131:395–401.

19. Meluzin J, Spinarova L, Bakala J, et al. Pulsed Doppler tissue imaging of the velocity of tricuspid annular systolic motion; a new, rapid, and noninvasive method of evaluating right ventricular systolic function. Eur Heart J 2001;22:340–8.

20. La Gerche A, Jurcut R, Voigt JU. Right ventricular function by strain echocardiography. Curr Opin Cardiol 2010;25:430–6.

21. Grapsa J, Dawson D, Nihoyannopoulos P. Assessment of right ventricular structure and function in pulmonary hypertension. J Cardiovasc Ultrasound 2011;19:115–25.

22. Duan YY, Harada K, Toyono M, et al. Effects of acute preload reduction on myocardial velocity during isovolumic contraction and myocardial acceleration in pediatric patients. Pediatr Cardiol 2006;27:32–6.

23. Teske AJ, De Boeck BW, Olimulder M, et al. Echocardiographic assessment of regional right ventricular function: a head-to-head comparison between 2-dimensional and tissue Doppler-derived strain analysis. J Am Soc Echocardiogr 2008;21:275–83.

24. Vitarelli A, Conde Y, Cimino E, et al. Assessment of right ventricular function by strain rate imaging in chronic obstructive pulmonary disease. Eur Respir J 2006;27:268–75.

25. Yeo TC, Dujardin KS, Tei C, et al. Value of a Doppler-derived index combining systolic and diastolic time intervals in predicting outcome in primary pulmonary hypertension. Am J Cardiol 1998;81:1157–61.

26. Jiang L, Siu SC, Handschumacher MD, et al. Three-dimensional echocardiography. In vivo validation for right ventricular volume and function. Circulation 1994;89:2342–50.

27. Lu X, Nadvoretskiy V, Bu L, et al. Accuracy and reproducibility of real-time three-dimensional echocardiography for assessment of right ventricular volumes and ejection fraction in children. J Am Soc Echocardiogr 2008;21:84–9.

28. Shiota T, Jones M, Chikada M, et al. Real-time three-dimensional echocardiography for determining right ventricular stroke volume in an animal model of chronic right ventricular volume overload. Circulation 1998;97:1897–900.

29. Liang XC, Cheung EW, Wong SJ, et al. Impact of right ventricular volume overload on three-dimensional global left ventricular mechanical dyssynchrony after surgical repair of tetralogy of Fallot. Am J Cardiol 2008;102:1731–6.

30. Ton-Nu TT, Levine RA, Handschumacher MD, et al. Geometric determinants of functional tricuspid regurgitation: insights from 3-dimensional echocardiography. Circulation 2006;114:143–9.

31. Pfisterer ME, Battler A, Zaret BL. Range of normal values for left and right ventricular ejection fraction at rest and during exercise assessed by radionuclide angiocardiography. Eur Heart J 1985;6:647–55.

32. Kjaer A, Lebech AM, Hesse B, et al. Right-sided cardiac function in healthy volunteers measured by first-pass radionuclide ventriculography and gated blood-pool SPECT: comparison with cine MRI. Clin Physiol Funct Imaging 2005;25:344–9.

33. Hesse B, Lindhardt TB, Acampa W, et al. EANM/ESC guidelines for radionuclide imaging of cardiac function. Eur J Nucl Med Mol Imaging 2008;35:851–85.

34. Hendel RC, Berman DS, Di Carli MF, et al. ACCF/ASNC/ACR/AHA/ASE/SCCT/SCMR/SNM 2009 appropriate use criteria for cardiac radionuclide imaging: a report of the American College of Cardiology Foundation Appropriate Use Criteria Task Force, the American Society of Nuclear Cardiology, the American College of Radiology, the American Heart Association, the American Society of Echocardiography, the Society of Cardiovascular Computed Tomography, the Society for Cardiovascular Magnetic Resonance, and the Society of Nuclear Medicine. Circulation 2009;119:e561–87.

35. Mielniczuk LM, Birnie D, Ziadi MC, et al. Relation between right ventricular function and increased right ventricular [18F]fluorodeoxyglucose accumulation in patients with heart failure. Circ Cardiovasc Imaging 2011;4:59–66.

36. Gomez A, Bialostozky D, Zajarias A, et al. Right ventricular ischemia in patients with primary pulmonary hypertension. J Am Coll Cardiol 2001;38:1137–42.

37. Bokhari S, Raina A, Rosenweig EB, et al. PET imaging may provide a novel biomarker and understanding of right ventricular dysfunction in patients with idiopathic pulmonary arterial hypertension. Circ Cardiovasc Imaging 2011;4:641–7.

38. Oikawa M, Kagaya Y, Otani H, et al. Increased [18F] fluorodeoxyglucose accumulation in right ventricular free wall in patients with pulmonary hypertension and the effect of epoprostenol. J Am Coll Cardiol 2005;45:1849–55.

39. James OG, Christensen JD, Wong TZ, et al. Utility of FDG PET/CT in inflammatory cardiovascular disease. Radiographics 2011;31:1271–86.

40. Youssef G, Beanlands RS, Birnie DH, et al. Cardiac sarcoidosis: applications of imaging in diagnosis and directing treatment. Heart 2011;97: 2078–87.

41. Gentzler RD 2nd, Briselli MF, Gault JH. Angiographic estimation of right ventricular volume in man. Circulation 1974;50:324–30.

42. Ferlinz J, Gorlin R, Cohn PF, et al. Right ventricular performance in patients with coronary artery disease. Circulation 1975;52:608–15.

43. Schoepf UJ, Goldhaber SZ, Costello P. Spiral computed tomography for acute pulmonary embolism. Circulation 2004;109:2160–7.

44. Schoepf UJ, Kucher N, Kipfmueller F, et al. Right ventricular enlargement on chest computed tomography: a predictor of early death in acute pulmonary embolism. Circulation 2004;110:3276–80.

45. Kang DK, Thilo C, Schoepf UJ, et al. CT signs of right ventricular dysfunction: prognostic role in acute pulmonary embolism. JACC Cardiovasc Imaging 2011;4:841–9.

46. Plumhans C, Muhlenbruch G, Rapaee A, et al. Assessment of global right ventricular function on 64-MDCT compared with MRI. AJR Am J Roentgenol 2008;190:1358–61.

47. Dogan H, Kroft LJ, Huisman MV, et al. Right ventricular function in patients with acute pulmonary embolism: analysis with electrocardiography-synchronized multi-detector row CT. Radiology 2007;242:78–84.

48. Taylor AJ, Cerqueira M, Hodgson JM, et al. ACCF/SCCT/ACR/AHA/ASE/ASNC/NASCI/SCAI/SCMR 2010 appropriate use criteria for cardiac computed tomography. A report of the American College of Cardiology Foundation Appropriate Use Criteria Task Force, the Society of Cardiovascular Computed Tomography, the American College of Radiology, the American Heart Association, the American Society of Echocardiography, the American Society of Nuclear Cardiology, the North American Society for Cardiovascular Imaging, the Society for Cardiovascular Angiography and Interventions, and the Society for Cardiovascular Magnetic Resonance. J Am Coll Cardiol 2010;56:1864–94.

49. Garcia-Alvarez A, Fernandez-Friera L, Lau JF, et al. Evaluation of right ventricular function and postoperative findings using cardiac computed tomography in patients with left ventricular assist devices. J Heart Lung Transplant 2011;30:896–903.

50. Cook SC, Dyke PC 2nd, Raman SV. Management of adults with congenital heart disease with cardiovascular computed tomography. J Cardiovasc Comput Tomogr 2008;2:12–22.

51. Bomma C, Dalal D, Tandri H, et al. Evolving role of multidetector computed tomography in evaluation of arrhythmogenic right ventricular dysplasia/cardiomyopathy. Am J Cardiol 2007;100:99–105.

52. Kim E, Choe YH, Han BK, et al. Right ventricular fat infiltration in asymptomatic subjects: observations from ECG-gated 16-slice multidetector CT. J Comput Assist Tomogr 2007;31:22–8.

53. Hendel RC, Patel MR, Kramer CM, et al. ACCF/ACR/SCCT/SCMR/ASNC/NASCI/SCAI/SIR 2006 appropriateness criteria for cardiac computed tomography and cardiac magnetic resonance imaging: a report of the American College of Cardiology Foundation Quality Strategic Directions Committee Appropriateness Criteria Working Group, American College of Radiology, Society of Cardiovascular Computed Tomography, Society for Cardiovascular Magnetic Resonance, American Society of Nuclear Cardiology, North American Society for Cardiac Imaging, Society for Cardiovascular Angiography and Interventions, and Society of Interventional Radiology. J Am Coll Cardiol 2006;48:1475–97.

54. Grothues F, Moon JC, Bellenger NG, et al. Interstudy reproducibility of right ventricular volumes, function, and mass with cardiovascular magnetic resonance. Am Heart J 2004;147:218–23.

55. Kuehne T, Yilmaz S, Steendijk P, et al. Magnetic resonance imaging analysis of right ventricular pressure-volume loops: in vivo validation and clinical application in patients with pulmonary hypertension. Circulation 2004;110:2010–6.

56. Saba TS, Foster J, Cockburn M, et al. Ventricular mass index using magnetic resonance imaging accurately estimates pulmonary artery pressure. Eur Respir J 2002;20:1519–24.

57. van Wolferen SA, Marcus JT, Boonstra A, et al. Prognostic value of right ventricular mass, volume, and function in idiopathic pulmonary arterial hypertension. Eur Heart J 2007;28:1250–7.

58. Fernandez-Friera L, Garcia-Alvarez A, Guzman G, et al. Apical right ventricular dysfunction in patients with pulmonary hypertension demonstrated with magnetic resonance. Heart 2011;97:1250–6.

59. Stevens GR, Garcia-Alvarez A, Sahni S, et al. Right ventricular dysfunction in pulmonary hypertension is independently related to pulmonary artery stiffness. JACC Cardiovasc Imaging 2012. [Epub ahead of print].

60. Moral S, Fernandez-Friera L, Stevens G, et al. New index alpha improves detection of pulmonary hypertension in comparison with other cardiac magnetic resonance indices. Int J Cardiol 2012. [Epub ahead of print].

61. Garcia-Alvarez A, Fernandez-Friera L, Mirelis JG, et al. Non-invasive estimation of pulmonary vascular resistance with cardiac magnetic resonance. Eur Heart J 2011;32:2438–45.

62. Sanz J, Garcia-Alvarez A, Fernandez-Friera L, et al. Right ventriculo-arterial coupling in pulmonary hypertension: a magnetic resonance study. Heart 2012;98(3):238–43.

63. Roeleveld RJ, Marcus JT, Faes TJ, et al. Interventricular septal configuration at MR imaging and pulmonary arterial pressure in pulmonary hypertension. Radiology 2005;234:710–7.

64. Dellegrottaglie S, Sanz J, Poon M, et al. Pulmonary hypertension: accuracy of detection with left ventricular septal-to-free wall curvature ratio measured at cardiac MR. Radiology 2007;243:63–9.

65. Sanz J, Dellegrottaglie S, Kariisa M, et al. Prevalence and correlates of septal delayed contrast enhancement in patients with pulmonary hypertension. Am J Cardiol 2007;100:731–5.

66. Tandri H, Castillo E, Ferrari VA, et al. Magnetic resonance imaging of arrhythmogenic right ventricular dysplasia: sensitivity, specificity, and observer variability of fat detection versus functional analysis of the right ventricle. J Am Coll Cardiol 2006;48: 2277–84.

67. Tandri H, Saranathan M, Rodriguez ER, et al. Noninvasive detection of myocardial fibrosis in arrhythmogenic right ventricular cardiomyopathy using delayed-enhancement magnetic resonance imaging. J Am Coll Cardiol 2005;45:98–103.

68. Marcus FI, McKenna WJ, Sherrill D, et al. Diagnosis of arrhythmogenic right ventricular cardiomyopathy/dysplasia: proposed modification of the task force criteria. Circulation 2010;121:1533–41.

69. Frank L, Dillman JR, Parish V, et al. Cardiovascular MR imaging of conotruncal anomalies. Radiographics 2010;30:1069–94.

70. Oosterhof T, van Straten A, Vliegen HW, et al. Preoperative thresholds for pulmonary valve replacement in patients with corrected tetralogy of Fallot using cardiovascular magnetic resonance. Circulation 2007;116:545–51.

71. Babu-Narayan SV, Kilner PJ, Li W, et al. Ventricular fibrosis suggested by cardiovascular magnetic resonance in adults with repaired tetralogy of Fallot and its relationship to adverse markers of clinical outcome. Circulation 2006;113: 405–13.

Right Ventricular Performance in Congenital Heart Disease: A Physiologic and Pathophysiologic Perspective

William E. Hopkins, MD

KEYWORDS

- Right ventricle • Congenital heart disease
- Eisenmeger syndrome • Pulmonary hypertension
- Pulmonary valve regurgitation

In cardiology, the predominant emphasis is on the left heart including the left ventricle and left atrium, mitral and aortic valves, and the coronary arteries. At times, it seems there is no attention paid to the right heart. I sometimes quip that most cardiologists do not even realize the heart has a right side! Because of success in the treatment of infants and children, the number of adults with congenital heart disease has greatly increased.[1–3] It is underappreciated that the right ventricle is often the primary determinant of long-term morbidity and mortality in patients with congenital heart disease.

When considering congenital heart disease, there are several fascinating questions related to the right ventricle. Extreme pressure load on the right ventricle in patients with acquired heart disease generally results in dilatation and failure of the right ventricle and premature death.[4–7] Why, then, do most adult patients with Eisenmenger physiology have normal right ventricular function and a better survival when compared with other patients with pulmonary hypertension despite the additional burdens of a cardiac defect, marked hypoxemia, and dramatic erythrocytosis?[8,9] Why does the right ventricle dilate in patients with a large atrial septal defect (ASD) but not in patients with a large ventricular septal defect (VSD)?[10–12] Why does the right ventricle dilate and sometimes fail in adult patients after surgical repair of Tetralogy of Fallot but almost never before surgical repair?[3,13,14]

A recent comprehensive review of the right ventricle in adult congenital heart disease was anomaly specific, comprehensive, and excellent.[13] Rather than emphasize specific anomalies, this article focuses on the unique physiology and pathophysiology found in patients with congenital heart disease.

PATHOPHYSIOLOGY: AN OVERVIEW

In acquired heart disease, one never considers the fetal cardiovascular system, the pulmonary valve, or the impact of a very low, pulmonary level left ventricular systolic pressure. Yet these and other anatomic and hemodynamic factors are important considerations in congenital heart disease. This

Conflict of interest: The author is on the Speaker's Bureau of Merck and Actelion.

Department of Medicine and Cardiology Unit, Pulmonary Hypertension and Adult Congenital Heart Disease Programs, Fletcher Allen Health Care, University of Vermont College of Medicine, McClure 1, MCHV Campus, 111 Colchester Avenue, Burlington, VT 05401, USA

E-mail address: william.hopkins@vtmednet.org

doi:10.1016/j.ccl.2012.03.006
0733-8651/12/$ – see front matter © 2012 Elsevier Inc. All rights reserved.

cardiology.theclinics.com

article focuses on six key physiologic and patho-physiologic concepts including:

1. Nonrestrictive hemodynamics and shunt physiology
2. The fetal cardiovascular system
3. Location of the cardiac anomaly relative to the tricuspid valve
4. Timing of the hemodynamic insult
5. The postoperative pulmonary valve
6. Left ventricular pressure and right ventricular performance.

It is the authors' hope that discussion of these physiologic and pathophysiologic concepts will lead to a better understanding of right ventricular performance in multiple different repaired and unrepaired congenital cardiac anomalies.

PATHOPHYSIOLOGY: NONRESTRICTIVE HEMODYNAMICS AND SHUNT PHYSIOLOGY
Overview

When considering the right ventricle in patients with congenital heart disease, one must understand the physiology and pathophysiology of shunt lesions. Excluding bicuspid aortic valves, shunts at the atrial, ventricular, or great artery level account for most patients with a congenital cardiac anomaly.[15] Shunt lesions that have the greatest impact on right ventricular performance (and left ventricular performance) are those that are hemodynamically nonrestrictive. In a general sense, a nonrestrictive defect or communication is large enough so that there is no pressure difference from one side of the defect or communication to the other. This concept is extremely important, so let us consider nonrestrictive hemodynamics at the atrial, ventricular, and great artery level.

PATHOPHYSIOLOGY: NONRESTRICTIVE HEMODYNAMICS AND SHUNT PHYSIOLOGY
"ASD Physiology"

Most texts list five anatomic types of ASDs: ostium secundum ASD, ostium primum ASD, superior sinus venosus defect, inferior sinus venosus defect, and coronary sinus type ASD (**Figs. 1**A and B).[10,11,16] Far and away, ostium secundum ASDs are the most common, followed by ostium

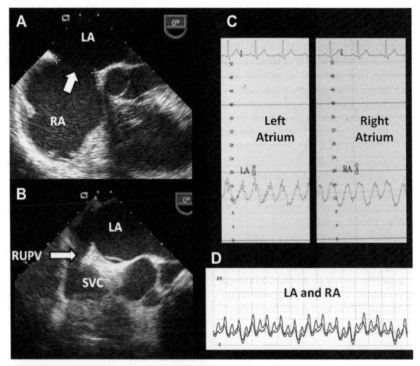

Fig. 1. Interatrial communications and nonrestrictive hemodynamics. (*A*) Transesophageal echocardiogram from an adult patient with an ostium secundum atrial septal defect. The arrow depicts the defect. (*B*) Transesophageal echocardiogram from an adult patient with a superior sinus venosus defect. Note the "connection" between the right upper pulmonary vein (*arrow*; RUPV) and the superior vena cava (SVC). This communication results in "ASD physiology." (*C* and *D*) Right and left atrial pressure tracings from a 29-year-old woman and a 52-year-old man with nonrestrictive ostium secundum atrial septal defects. (*C*) The catheter was pulled back from the left atrium to the right atrium. (*D*) The pressure tracings were recorded simultaneously. LA, left atrium; RA, right atrium.

primum ASD and superior sinus venosus defect. Inferior sinus venosus defects and coronary sinus type ASD are unusual or even rare. It has been brilliantly argued that sinus venosus defects are not a true ASD but result secondary to abnormal venous development (unroofing of the superior or inferior right pulmonary veins).[17] Further, coronary sinus type ASD result secondary to unroofing of the coronary sinus with the normal os of the coronary sinus "serving" as the communication between the left and right atria. Given these anatomic and developmental considerations, it is probably better to refer to these defects overall as "interatrial communications" rather than ASD. More important to this discussion is that all these patients exhibit what I often refer to as "ASD physiology" and the ultimate effect on the right ventricle is indistinguishable between the defects. The anatomy of the interatrial communication is important to the surgeon, but not to the right ventricle! To better understand this, one needs to understand nonrestrictive physiology at the level of the atria.

A nonrestrictive defect at the atrial level is characterized by equal pressure in the right and left atria throughout the cardiac cycle (see **Figs. 1C** and D).[10,12,16] This is the case independent of the anatomic type of interatrial communication. Stated another way, in patients with a nonrestrictive defect at the atrial level, there is no pressure drop from one atrial chamber to the other. Consequently, atrial pressure does not determine the magnitude or direction of shunt in patients with "ASD physiology." Instead, in patients with a nonrestrictive atrial communication, it is the relative compliance of the right and left ventricles that determines the magnitude and direction of shunt.[10,11,16,18] In most cases, compliance of the right ventricle is far greater than the compliance of the left ventricle and the resultant shunt is left-to-right with volume loading of the right heart (see later discussion).

PATHOPHYSIOLOGY: NONRESTRICTIVE HEMODYNAMICS AND SHUNT PHYSIOLOGY
Ventricular and Great Artery Level Shunts

This article does not focus on a detailed discussion of the anatomic types of VSDs but, instead, focuses on physiology and pathophysiology. A nonrestrictive defect at the ventricular level is characterized by equal pressure in the right and left ventricles throughout the cardiac cycle (**Figs. 2A and B**).[12,19–21] This is true whether the defect

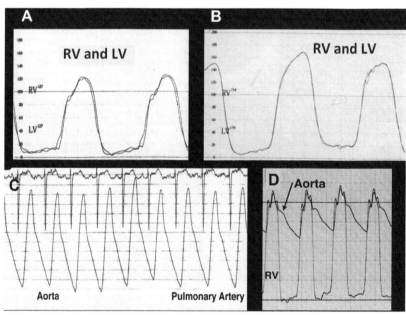

Fig. 2. Nonrestrictive hemodynamics: post-tricuspid defects. (*A*) Simultaneous pressure tracings from the right and left ventricles of a 40-year-old man with a nonrestrictive perimembranous ventricular septal defect and Eisenmenger syndrome. (*B*) Simultaneous pressure tracings from the right and left ventricles of a 35-year-old woman with unrepaired tetralogy of Fallot and Down syndrome. (*C*) Simultaneous pressure tracings from the aorta and pulmonary artery of a 20-year-old woman with a nonrestrictive patent ductus arteriosus and Eisenmenger syndrome. The catheter was pulled from the aorta to the pulmonary artery via the ductus arteriosus. (*D*) Simultaneous pressure tracings from the right ventricle and aorta of a 25-year-old woman with truncus arteriosus and Eisenmenger syndrome. LV, left ventricle; RV, right ventricle.

is an isolated VSD (perimembranous or muscular) or associated with more complex anomalies that feature a VSD such as Tetralogy of Fallot, complete atrioventricular canal defects, transposition of the great arteries with VSD, truncus arteriosus, and double outlet right ventricle (**Fig. 3**). In fact, the VSD is physiologically nonrestrictive in virtually all patients with these complex anomalies. In all patients with a nonrestrictive VSD, the pulmonary artery and aortic systolic pressure are also equal unless there is associated outflow obstruction (ie, Tetralogy of Fallot).

In patients with a nonrestrictive defect at the great artery level, such as a patent ductus arteriosus (PDA) or aortopulmonary window, pulmonary artery and aortic pressures are equal throughout the cardiac cycle as is right and left ventricular systolic pressure (see **Fig. 2**C).[12,19,20,22,23]

In patients with nonrestrictive defects at both the ventricular and great artery level, such as truncus arteriosus, pressure is equal in the right and left ventricles throughout the cardiac cycle and equal in the pulmonary artery and aorta throughout the cardiac cycle (see **Fig. 2**D). Similarly, in patients with nonrestrictive defects at both the atrial and ventricular level, such as a complete atrioventricular canal defect, pressure is equal in the right and left atrium throughout the cardiac cycle, equal in the right and left ventricle throughout the cardiac cycle, and equal in the aorta and pulmonary artery during systole (see **Fig. 3**D).

Concentrating on physiology and pathophysiology, by definition, patients with a hemodynamically nonrestrictive defect at the level of the ventricles, great arteries, or both have systemic level right ventricular pressure (see **Fig. 2**). Put another way, the right ventricles of these patients are under an extreme pressure load. This is independent of the anatomic type of defect. Because it is equal in the two ventricles, pressure does not determine the magnitude or direction of shunt.

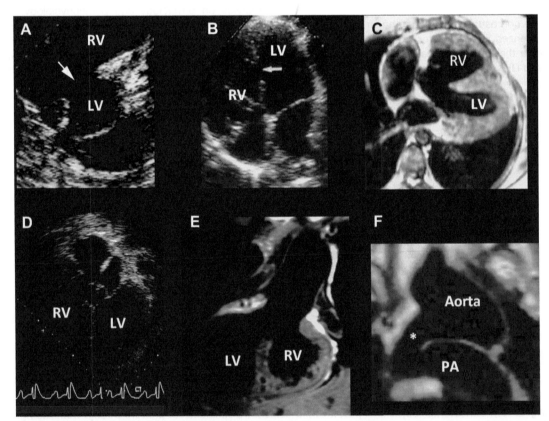

Fig. 3. Nonrestrictive post-tricuspid defects. (*A*) Perimembranous ventricular septal defect (*arrow*) and Eisenmenger syndrome. (*B*) Midmuscular ventricular septal defect (*arrow*) and Eisenmenger syndrome. (*C*) Tetralogy of Fallot and pulmonary atresia. (*D*) Complete atrioventricular canal defect and Eisenmenger syndrome. (*E*) Congenitally corrected transposition with a ventricular septal defect. Note the ventricular inversion. The patient also had high-grade pulmonary valve stenosis and "tetralogy of Fallot physiology." (*F*) Patent ductus arteriosus (*asterisk*) and Eisenmenger syndrome. All images were from adult patients. (*A*, *B*, and *D*) echocardiograms; (*C*, *E*, and *F*) MRIs. LV, left ventricle; PA, pulmonary artery; RV, right ventricle.

Rather, the relative "resistance" in the pulmonary and systemic vascular beds (± an anatomic obstruction) is the determinant (see later discussion).

Hemodynamically restrictive defects at the atrial, ventricular, or great artery level are smaller and rarely result in a significant volume and/or pressure load on the right ventricle. Restrictive defects are not considered in this article.

PATHOPHYSIOLOGY: THE FETAL CARDIOVASCULAR SYSTEM

To understand why right ventricular performance can be so dramatically different in patients with acquired and congenital heart disease, one needs to understand the fetal cardiovascular system. Hypoxemia, a low-resistance systemic circulation, a high-resistance pulmonary circulation, a ductus arteriosus, a ductus venosus, and right-to-left flow across the foreman ovale characterize the normal fetal heart and circulation. In addition, both the lungs and kidneys receive very little flow during fetal life, but they are intimately tied together as amniotic fluid consists primarily of fetal urine and an adequate amount of amniotic fluid is essential for normal maturation of the fetal lungs. The fetal circulation has been described as a "shunt dependent circulation."[24,25]

Most people that have spent even a small amount of time considering the fetal cardiovascular system understand that it is "designed" to shunt blood returning from the placenta via the umbilical vein across the foreman ovale to the left heart to enhance oxygen delivery to the heart and brain. However, what is not appreciated by most people is that the normal fetus lives at a very low oxygen tension as even the blood in the left atrium, left ventricle, and ascending aorta is extremely hypoxemic with a saturation of about 65%.[24,25] Further, most people understand the role of the ductus arteriosus, but few people realize that, in the normal fetus, the ductus arteriosus is large and hemodynamically nonrestrictive. Therefore, in the normal fetal circulation, pressure in the fetal pulmonary artery and aorta is equal throughout the cardiac cycle as is systolic right and left ventricular pressure (**Fig. 4**A).[25] The result is that the right and left ventricular free wall thickness and force development are equal throughout fetal development and the interventricular septum is midline between the ventricular chambers and flat throughout the cardiac cycle (see **Figs. 4**B and C).[19,20,26] Contractile function in the fetal right ventricle is characterized by circumferential fiber shortening similar to that of the mature left ventricle. This means the normal fetal heart has systemic level pulmonary and right ventricular pressure. Put another way, we all had severe pulmonary hypertension at one point in our lives! Despite a systemic level pressure load, fetal right ventricular function is normal. This

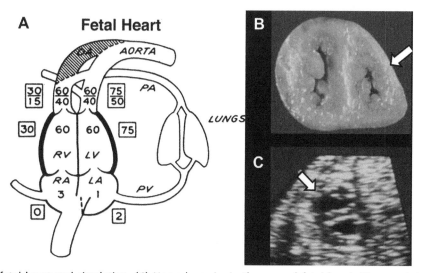

Fig. 4. The fetal heart and circulation. (*A*) Hemodynamics in the normal fetal heart. The equal right and left ventricular systolic pressure is secondary to the nonrestrictive ductus arteriosus. The numbers in the boxes outside the heart are postnatal pressures. (*B*) Postmortem specimen from a 25-week fetus that died in utero from noncardiac complications. The heart was morphologically normal. (*C*) Echocardiogram from a normal 20-week fetus. In both panels, the arrow points to the right ventricle. Note the equal thickness of the right and left ventricular free walls. Note also the striking similarity of the normal fetal heart to the hearts with nonrestrictive post-tricuspid defects in **Fig. 6**. ([*A*] *From* Rudolph AM. The changes in the circulation after birth. Their importance in congenital heart disease. Circulation 1970;41:343–59; with permission.)

has tremendous implications for the fate of the right ventricle in many patients born with a congenital heart defect (see later discussion).

PATHOPHYSIOLOGY: PRE-TRICUSPID VERSUS POST-TRICUSPID DEFECTS
Overview

What is the impact of fetal cardiovascular physiology on hearts with nonrestrictive shunt lesions? This impact depends greatly on whether the defect and resultant shunt is proximal to the tricuspid valve (pre-tricuspid defects) or distal to the tricuspid valve (post-tricuspid defects). Patients with nonrestrictive pre-tricuspid defects are characterized by volume-loaded, dilated right ventricles, whereas patients with nonrestrictive post-tricuspid defects are characterized by pressure-loaded, hypertrophied right ventricles and a heart that more closely resembles a normal fetal heart than it does a typical child or adult heart (**Figs. 5** and **6**).

At birth, the pulmonary vascular resistance precipitously decreases but only to systemic level. The muscular pulmonary arteries present in fetal and newborn lungs then mature over the course of weeks.[25] With maturation and remodeling come a fall in pulmonary vascular resistance. The mature pulmonary vasculature can vasodilate and accommodate large increases in flow without a significant increase in pressure. Maturation of the pulmonary circulation is accompanied by a fall in right ventricular systolic pressure and regression of right ventricular wall thickness. Over

the course of weeks to months, the right ventricle remodels into a thin-walled, crescent-shaped chamber with longitudinal fiber shortening during systole.[25,27]

Pre-tricuspid Defects

As discussed above, the relative compliance of the right and left ventricles determines the magnitude and direction of shunt in patients with nonrestrictive ASD physiology. Therefore, patients with nonrestrictive pre-tricuspid defects do not manifest any significant shunt until the pulmonary vasculature matures, the right ventricular wall thickness regresses, and right ventricular compliance increases—a process that may take months. Because significant left-to-right shunt is delayed until the pulmonary vasculature has matured, patients with nonrestrictive ASD physiology typically have a normal pulmonary artery pressure despite high-volume flow in the pulmonary arteries. Patients are characterized by a dilated, volume-loaded right ventricle generally with normal systolic function for many decades (see **Fig. 5**A). The onset of pulmonary hypertension is typically delayed for many decades and is more often modest in magnitude.[28] Significant pulmonary and right ventricular hypertension leads to further dilatation of the right ventricle and, often, associated right ventricular systolic dysfunction. If the pulmonary hypertension is severe (atypical in patients with nonrestrictive ASD physiology), the right ventricle will fail and the left-to-right shunt will reverse and become right-to-left (Eisenmenger physiology) (see **Fig. 5**B).[12] Survival in these

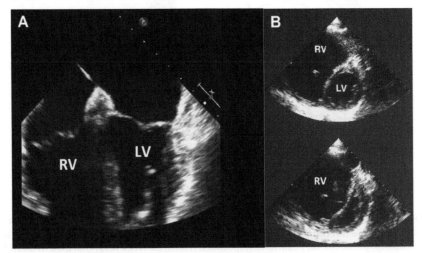

Fig. 5. Interatrial communications and volume-loaded right ventricle. (A) Transesophageal echocardiogram from a 52-year-old man with an ostium secundum atrial septal defect and a pulmonary to systemic flow ratio of ~2 (Q_p:Q_s). Pulmonary artery pressure was normal. (B) Transthoracic echocardiographic parasternal short-axis images from an adult patient with a nonrestrictive superior sinus venosus defect and severe pulmonary arterial hypertension with Eisenmenger physiology. LV, left ventricle; RV, right ventricle.

patients is better compared with patients with idiopathic pulmonary arterial hypertension and other forms of pulmonary hypertension because of the atrial communication that allows for right-to-left shunt, preserved filling of the left ventricle, and a better cardiac output.[8–11] Although severe pulmonary hypertension is uncommon in patients with ASD physiology, older adults with nonrestrictive interatrial communications are still characterized by an increased incidence of heart failure and atrial fibrillation, and by reduced survival.[10,11,28–30] In fact, little appreciated is that ASD physiology volume loads the pulmonary veins and left atrium in addition to the right heart. This is likely the reason for the high incidence of atrial fibrillation in older patients with an interatrial communication (repaired or unrepaired) and the reason that an isolated right-sided maze procedure does not decrease this incidence.[31]

Post-tricuspid Defects

The pathophysiology is markedly different in patients born with a nonrestrictive defect distal to the tricuspid valve (post-tricuspid defects). This includes patients with nonrestrictive defects at the ventricular level or nonrestrictive defects at the great artery level. At birth and beyond, right and left ventricular systolic pressure remains equal—continuing the fetal relationship, as discussed above (see **Fig. 6**).

Large left-to-right shunts are characteristic of infants born with nonrestrictive post-tricuspid defects and no anatomic obstruction to right ventricular outflow. The magnitude of the shunt is not determined by a pressure difference between the left and right ventricles in patients with a nonrestrictive VSD or between the aorta and pulmonary artery in patients with a nonrestrictive PDA but by

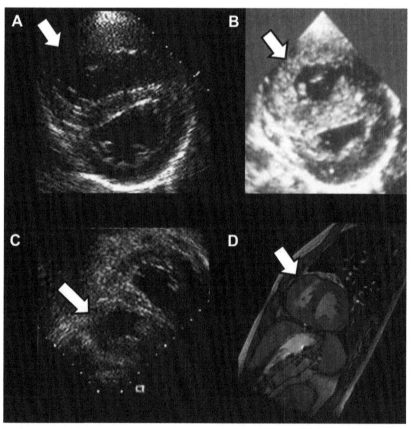

Fig. 6. Nonrestrictive post-tricuspid defects: ventricular morphology. (*A*) Transthoracic echocardiographic parasternal short-axis image from a 14-year-old girl with a nonrestrictive perimembranous ventricular septal defect and Eisenmenger syndrome. (*B*) Transthoracic echocardiographic parasternal short-axis image from a 29-year-old man with truncus arteriosus and Eisenmenger syndrome. (*C*) Transthoracic echocardiographic subcostal short-axis image from a 77-year-old woman with a perimembranous ventricular septal defect and Eisenmenger syndrome. (*D*) MRI from a 42-year-old man with unrepaired tetralogy of Fallot and pulmonary atresia. In all four panels, the arrow depicts the right ventricle. In each patient, the interventricular septum is flat and the thickness of the right and left ventricular free walls are the same. Note the similarity to the normal fetal heart depicted in **Fig. 4**.

the relative "resistance" of the pulmonary and systemic vascular beds. In infants with nonrestrictive VSD, the large shunt volume loads the "noncompliant" left and right ventricles and in infants with nonrestrictive PDA, the large shunt volume loads the "noncompliant" left ventricle. In both circumstances, systemic circulation is decreased and the infants are characterized by congestion and failure to thrive.[21,22] If left unrepaired, the infant suffers one of two fates: death (secondary to failure to thrive) or Eisenmenger syndrome. An occlusive vasculopathy in the small pulmonary arteries and arterioles, or what the author refers to as the "Eisenmenger reaction," is life saving because the volume of the left-to-right shunt decreases proportional to the increase in resistance in the pulmonary vascular bed.[12,21,22] This facilitates greater systemic blood flow and improved well-being of the infant. This "Eisenmenger reaction" begins in the first year of life.[32] Unfortunately, it advances such that a progressive occlusive vasculopathy with plexiform lesions develops and pulmonary vascular resistance ultimately increases to or greater than systemic vascular resistance. The result is the full blown Eisenmenger syndrome with reversal of the shunt to right-to-left, hypoxemia, and erythrocytosis.[12,21,22,33,34] Patients with defects at the ventricular level are characterized by clubbing and cyanosis of the upper and lower extremity digits, whereas patients with a PDA are characterized by differential clubbing and cyanosis, that is, clubbing and cyanosis of the toes but not the fingers.

In those patients with nonrestrictive post-tricuspid defects that are not surgically repaired and survive with Eisenmenger physiology, right ventricular wall thickness does not regress. With aging and growth, right ventricular wall thickness increases at a rate equal to that of the left ventricle and the thickness of the right and left ventricular free walls remains equal.[19,20] Right and left ventricular wall thickness are equal as a fetus, during infancy in the left-to-right shunt or pre-Eisenmenger phase, and during adolescence and adulthood in the Eisenmenger phase. The interventricular septum does not bow into the right ventricle but remains in the midline between the ventricular chambers and flat throughout the cardiac cycle (see **Fig. 6**). The anatomy of hearts with a nonrestrictive post-tricuspid defect more closely resembles a normal fetal heart than it does a typical child or adult heart (see **Figs. 4** and **6**). This fetal morphology persists for as long as the nonrestrictive post-tricuspid defect is present. Normal right ventricular function is the rule rather than the exception in these patients despite severe systemic level pulmonary and right ventricular hypertension, hypoxemia, and erythrocytosis. Survival is greater than all other patients with severe pulmonary hypertension and even greater than survival after lung transplantation.[8,9,20,35]

When the right ventricle fails in patients with a nonrestrictive post-tricuspid defect, it does so in proportion to the left ventricle. In a previous study, we reported a linear relationship between right and left ventricular systolic function, which suggests that the two ventricles function as a "common ventricular unit"[19] and are equally vulnerable to perturbations that affect ventricular contractile function. Of 50 adolescents and adults with Eisenmenger syndrome and post-tricuspid defects, seven had significant right and left ventricular systolic dysfunction. Six of the seven had additional loads on the ventricles such as valvular heart disease (truncal valve insufficiency or stenosis in truncus arteriosus or atrioventricular valve regurgitation in common atrioventricular canal defects), iron deficiency, or both.[19] The most common cause of death in patients with Eisenmenger syndrome is not heart failure or sudden arrhythmic death. Rather, it seems to be sudden death secondary to intrapulmonary hemorrhage or rupture of a dilated pulmonary trunk.[35]

As long as there is a nonrestrictive post-tricuspid defect, this "fetal morphology" will be present even if there is associated obstruction to right ventricular outflow (tetralogy of Fallot, transposition of the great arteries with VSD and pulmonic stenosis), associated obstruction to left ventricular outflow (aortic stenosis, interrupted aortic arch, or coarctation of the aorta), or associated obstruction to right and left ventricular outflow (truncus arteriosus with truncal valve stenosis) (see **Figs. 2** and **6**). The presence of an obstruction does not affect the relationship of the right and left ventricles; it affects only the magnitude and direction of shunt. Infants and children with tetralogy of Fallot do not die because of failure of a pressure-loaded right ventricle but rather from severe hypoxemia related to right ventricular outflow obstruction and inadequate pulmonary blood flow (see later discussion).

If there is also a volume load at the ventricular level, such as truncal valve regurgitation in patients with unrepaired truncus arteriosus or atrioventricular valve regurgitation in patients with complete atrioventricular canal defects, it will be "shared" by both ventricles. The fundamental relationship between the right and left ventricles is not altered—pressure and wall thickness are equal. As pointed out above, an additional load on both ventricles may predispose to failure of both ventricles and premature death.[19,35]

PATHOPHYSIOLOGY: TIMING OF THE HEMODYNAMIC INSULT

It is all about timing! Extreme pressure load on the right ventricle in patients with acquired heart disease generally results in dilatation and failure of the right ventricle and premature death.[4–8] The typical child or adult that develops significant pulmonary hypertension does so after an interval of normal right heart hemodynamics characterized by low pulmonary artery and right ventricular systolic pressures. Their right ventricle is not suited to withstand the elevated pressure load present in severe pulmonary hypertension. In patients with severe pulmonary hypertension, it is right ventricular failure that is most often the cause of premature death.[4–8]

In contrast, despite the extreme pressure load, in patients with nonrestrictive post-tricuspid defects, the right ventricle typically maintains normal function for a lifetime. This is despite the additional burdens hypoxemia and erythrocytosis (Eisenmenger syndrome or "tetralogy of Fallot physiology"). The reason is that the right ventricle of these patients never remodeled. They never had a low pressure interval during which re-modeling occurred. Patients born with a non-restrictive post-tricuspid defect are primed and ready for the systemic level right ventricular pressure load as it represents a continuation of fetal hemodynamics with systemic-level right ventricular pressure.

So what happens to the right ventricles of patients who had a nonrestrictive post-tricuspid defect who undergo surgical repair and subsequently develop significant pulmonary and right ventricular hypertension? Do their right ventricles avoid the ultimate fate of failure and death? The answer is no! As long as the systolic pressure falls to a normal or near-normal range following surgical repair, right ventricular wall thickness will regress, compliance will increase, and a crescent-shaped right ventricular chamber will result. Patients that subsequently develop significant pulmonary hypertension suffer the same fate as patients with idiopathic pulmonary arterial hypertension, right ventricular failure, and premature death.[8] Similarly, occasional patients with a small restrictive VSD and normal right ventricular systolic pressure develop intracavitary right ventricular outflow obstruction ("double-chamber right ventricle"). If significant enough, the right ventricle of these patients will dilate and fail.[36] The remodeled right ventricle rarely does well when faced with a significant pressure load—no matter its history!

PATHOPHYSIOLOGY: THE POSTOPERATIVE PULMONARY VALVE

Acquired pulmonary valve disease is extremely uncommon. Significant regurgitation has been reported in some patients with metastatic carcinoid syndrome and significant stenosis in some patients following a Ross procedure for aortic stenosis.[37–39] Interestingly, the pulmonary valve is virtually always spared in rheumatic valvular disease and it seems to be spared in anorexigen-induced valvular disease.[40,41] I have cared for one patient who developed severe pulmonary valve stenosis secondary to radiation therapy for childhood cancer. I have seen multiple hundreds of patients with severe pulmonary hypertension, but have yet to identify significant pulmonary valve regurgitation in any of these patients. I would go so far as to say that most cardiologists rarely consider the pulmonary valve in their day-to-day practice. So why devote any attention to the pulmonary valve, let alone an entire section of this article? The reason is that the pulmonary valve is an important determinant of long-term right ventricular "health" in patients with congenital heart disease. This article primarily focuses on regurgitation rather than stenosis.

Tetralogy of Fallot is a fascinating congenital anomaly that has received a great deal of attention in both its native state and in the postoperative setting. Tetralogy hearts are characterized by a VSD, right ventricular outflow obstruction, right ventricular hypertrophy, and an overriding aorta. Rarely mentioned is that the VSD in patients with tetralogy is nonrestrictive with equalization of right and left ventricular pressure (see **Fig. 2**B).[42] Right ventricular hypertrophy occurs because the load on the right ventricle is identical to that on the left ventricle and wall thickness is equal in the two chambers—similar to that described in patients with a VSD or PDA and Eisenmenger syndrome (see **Fig. 6**D). Premature death is common in patients with tetralogy of Fallot, but not because of right ventricular failure.[42] Surgical repair of this defect has been extremely successful with an excellent long-term survival.[43]

Surgical repair of tetralogy of Fallot includes closure of the VSD and relief of right ventricular outflow obstruction. Most often, right ventricular systolic pressure falls to normal or near normal. The right ventricle remodels with regression of wall thickness. However, the surgical correction of tetralogy of Fallot often disrupts the pulmonary valve. A high proportion of these patients develop significant pulmonary valve regurgitation with chronic regurgitant fractions of 50% or greater. Preoperative pressure load, which is hemodynamically well tolerated, is replaced by volume overload of the right ventricle and chamber dilatation (**Fig. 7**). The volume load is generally well tolerated for decades but it can lead to exertional dyspnea secondary to a diminished cardiac output, right ventricular failure (in some cases), and an increased incidence of atrial and ventricular arrhythmias. Accordingly, there has been a great deal of focus on the right ventricle and pulmonary valve, including consideration of pulmonary valve replacement in postoperative tetralogy patients.[3,13,14,44–52] Similar pathophysiology is found in some patients following repair of isolated pulmonary valve stenosis—especially following surgical repair.[13,53,54] Although these patients are less likely to have the arrhythmic complications of postoperative tetralogy patients, at a minimum, they warrant lifetime surveillance of their right ventricles.

It is important to emphasize that pulmonary artery hypertension in patients with severe pulmonary valve regurgitation can increase the magnitude of regurgitation and, therefore, increase the volume load on the dilated right ventricle (see later discussion).

PATHOPHYSIOLOGY: LEFT VENTRICULAR PRESSURE AND RIGHT VENTRICULAR PERFORMANCE

The final pathophysiologic consideration is the impact of left ventricular pressure on right ventricular performance. In this section, the impact of a very low left ventricular systolic pressure is considered (for left ventricular diastolic pressure, see later discussion).

It is already emphasized that the right ventricle typically does not fail when systemic level pressure is present from birth. Because of the unique physiology of the fetal circulation, the right ventricle is primed and ready for this extreme pressure load. Contractile function is preserved and, importantly, competence of the tricuspid valve is the rule rather than the exception. However, a group of patients with congenital heart disease has systemic level right ventricular pressure from birth. Still, right ventricular dilatation and failure is a significant long-term concern.[55–58]

Patients with congenitally corrected transposition of the great arteries (ventricular inversion) and patients with complete transposition of the great arteries and a Mustard or Senning atrial baffle also have systemic-level right ventricular pressure from birth. However, unlike patients with a nonrestrictive post-tricuspid defect and Eisenmenger physiology or tetralogy of Fallot, the right ventricle is "connected" to the aorta and functions as the systemic ventricle in patients with these transposition complexes (**Fig. 8**A). These patients are also characterized by a left ventricle that is "connected" to the pulmonary circulation. With maturation of the pulmonary vasculature, left ventricular systolic pressure falls to levels characteristic of the "pulmonary" ventricle. The left ventricle myocardium regresses and the interventricular septum bows into the left ventricular chamber (see **Figs. 8**A and B). This

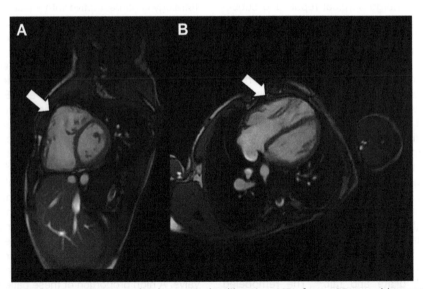

Fig. 7. Pulmonary valve regurgitation and right ventricular dilatation. MRIs from a 35-year-old man with a history of tetralogy of Fallot status after repair in early childhood. The patient has severe pulmonary valve regurgitation with a regurgitant fraction of ~70%. The arrow points to the dilated, volume-loaded right ventricle in both panels.

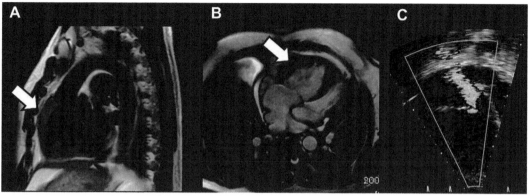

Fig. 8. Transposition complexes. (A) and (B) MRIs from a 35-year-old man with complete transposition of the great arteries and a Mustard atrial baffle. The arrow points to the morphologic right ventricle. Note the bowing of the interventricular septum into the left ventricle, the decreased wall thickness of the morphologic left ventricle compared with the morphologic right ventricle, and the origin of the aorta from the morphologic right ventricle (panel A). (C) Transthoracic echocardiogram from a 25-year-old man also with complete transposition of the great arteries and a Mustard atrial baffle. Color Doppler depicts significant tricuspid regurgitation.

anatomic and hemodynamic relationship persists in patients with complete transposition of the great arteries and a Mustard or Senning atrial baffle but not in those with complete transposition of the great arteries who had an arterial switch procedure. The right ventricle is also the high-pressure systemic ventricle in patients with congenitally corrected transposition and an intact ventricular septum, as well as in patients that underwent a classic repair of an associated VSD with or without pulmonary valve stenosis.[55,56]

In patients with one of these transposition complexes, the interventricular septum shifts toward the left ventricle. This septal shift can distort the tricuspid annulus and result in significant tricuspid valve regurgitation with the addition of a volume load to the pressure-loaded right ventricle (see **Fig. 8**C). Modern surgical techniques, such as the arterial switch operation for complete transposition of the great arteries and the "double switch" procedure for patients with congenitally corrected transposition and a nonrestrictive VSD, reestablishes the morphologic left ventricle as the systemic ventricle and the morphologic right ventricle as the venous ventricle.[57,58] Although it has been stated that the tricuspid valve is not suited to high pressures, if the annulus does not dilate, as in patients with nonrestrictive post-tricuspid defects, tricuspid regurgitation is rarely a significant issue.

Therapeutics and Prevention

As discussed above, patients with interatrial communications (pre-tricuspid defects) are characterized, not only by a volume-loaded, dilated right ventricle, but also by dilated pulmonary veins and atria.[10,11,31] Interatrial communications should be closed to enhance survival and reduce the incidence of heart failure and atrial fibrillation.[10,11,28–31] Ostium secundum atrial septal defects can often be closed with a percutaneous closure device, but the other anatomic types of interatrial communications have to be closed via an open surgical procedure.[11] The primary contraindication to closure of an interatrial communication is significant, especially severe pulmonary arterial hypertension. Patients with interatrial communications and severe pulmonary arterial hypertension, especially those associated with Eisenmenger physiology, have an increased surgical mortality and worse clinical outcome than those in whom the defect remains open.[8,10,11] The presence of an interatrial communication in patients with severe pulmonary arterial hypertension allows for better filling of the left ventricle and a better systemic cardiac output.

Despite a significantly greater longevity compared with all other patients with severe pulmonary hypertension, survival is still far from normal in adults with Eisenmenger syndrome. Exciting new data suggests that patients with Eisenmenger physiology benefit from advanced medical therapy for their pulmonary arterial hypertension.[59–63]

Patients with congenital heart disease and volume-loaded, dilated right ventricles are especially vulnerable to the deleterious effects of left ventricular diastolic dysfunction. This is important to note in the current era when inactivity and obesity are common. Obesity, obstructive sleep apnea, systemic hypertension, and diabetes mellitus all promote left ventricular diastolic dysfunction, increased left atrial pressure, and ultimately increased pulmonary artery pressure. In patients with a nonrestrictive interatrial communication, decreased left ventricular compliance increases the magnitude of the left-to-right shunt and further decreases systemic cardiac output.[11] Elevation of the pulmonary artery pressure increases the magnitude of pulmonary valve regurgitation and the load on the right ventricle in patients after repair of tetralogy of Fallot or isolated pulmonary valve stenosis. The result is a further decrease in cardiac output, increased dyspnea, and an increased likelihood of right ventricular failure. Maintaining as low a left atrial pressure as possible will promote forward, rather than backward, blood flow in these patients. Patients with congenital heart disease should adhere to a lifetime of exercise, weight control, and salt restriction. Instead, inactivity and obesity are common.

SUMMARY

Right ventricular performance in patients with congenital heart disease depends on a unique set of physiologic and pathophysiologic factors that are rarely considered in acquired heart disease. The ultimate fate of the right ventricle in these patients depends on nonrestrictive shunt physiology, the location of the primary anomaly relative to the tricuspid valve, the timing of the hemodynamic insult, the competence of the often forgotten pulmonary valve, and the left ventricular pressure in both systole and diastole. At times, the result is a heart that more closely resembles a normal fetal heart than a typical child or adult heart.

REFERENCES

1. Perloff JK. Historical perspective. In: Perloff JK, Child JS, editors. Congenital heart disease in adults. 2nd edition. Philadelphia: W.B. Saunders; 1998. p. 3–8.
2. Gatzoulis MA, Webb GD. Adults with congenital heart disease: a growing population. In: Gatzoulis MA, Webb GD, editors. Diagnosis and management of adult congenital heart disease. New York: Churchill Livingstone; 2003. p. 3–6.
3. Warnes CA. The adult with congenital heart disease: born to be bad? J Am Coll Cardiol 2005;46:1–8.
4. Fuster V, Steele PM, Edwards WD, et al. Primary pulmonary hypertension: natural history and the importance of thrombosis. Circulation 1984;70:580–7.
5. D'Alonzo GE, Barst RJ, Ayres SM, et al. Survival in patients with primary pulmonary hypertension. Results from a national prospective registry. Ann Intern Med 1991;115:343–9.
6. McLaughlin VV, Presberg KW, Doyle RL, et al. Prognosis of pulmonary arterial hypertension: ACCP evidence-based clinical practice guidelines. Chest 2004;126:78S–92S.
7. Benza RL, Miller DP, Gromberg-Maitland M, et al. Predicting survival in pulmonary arterial hypertension: insights from the Registry to Evaluate Early and Long-Term Pulmonary Arterial Hypertension Disease Management (REVEAL). Circulation 2010; 122:164–72.
8. Hopkins WE, Ochoa LL, Richardson GW, et al. Comparison of the hemodynamics and survival of adults with severe primary pulmonary hypertension or Eisenmenger syndrome. J Heart Lung Transplant 1996;15:100–5.
9. Saha A, Balakrishnan KG, Ja-iswal PK, et al. Prognosis for patients with Eisenmenger syndrome of various aetiology. Int J Cardiol 1994;45:199–207.
10. Hopkins WE. Atrial septal defect. Curr Treat Options Cardiovasc Med 1999;1:301–10.
11. Webb G, Gatzoulis MA. Atrial septal defects in the adult: recent progress and overview. Circulation 2006;114:1645–53.
12. Hopkins WE. Severe pulmonary hypertension in congenital heart disease: a review of Eisenmenger syndrome. Curr Opin Cardiol 1995;10:517–23.
13. Warnes CA. Adult congenital heart disease: importance of the right ventricle. J Am Coll Cardiol 2009; 54:1903–10.
14. Frigiola A, Redington AN, Cullen S, et al. Pulmonary regurgitation is an important determinant of right ventricular contractile dysfunction in patients with surgically repaired tetralogy of Fallot. Circulation 2004;110(Suppl 2):153–7.
15. Hoffman JIE, Kaplan S. The incidence of congenital heart disease. J Am Coll Cardiol 2002;39: 1890–900.
16. Perloff JK. Atrial septal defect: simple and complex. In: Perloff JK, editor. Clinical recognition of congenital heart disease. 5th edition. Philadelphia: Saunders; 2003. p. 233–99.
17. Van Praagh SV, Carrera ME, Sanders SP, et al. Sinus venosus defects: unroofing of the right pulmonary veins—anatomic and echocardiographic findings and surgical treatment. Am Heart J 1994;128:365–79.
18. Rowe GG, Castilo CA, Maxwell GM, et al. Atrial septal defect and the mechanism of shunt. Am Heart J 1961;61:369–74.
19. Hopkins WE, Waggoner AD. Severe pulmonary hypertension without right ventricular failure: the unique hearts of patients with Eisenmenger syndrome. Am J Cardiol 2002;89:34–8.
20. Hopkins WE. The remarkable right ventricle of patients with Eisenmenger syndrome. Coron Artery Dis 2005;16:19–25.
21. Perloff JK. Ventricular septal defect. In: Perloff JK, editor. Clinical recognition of congenital heart disease. 5th edition. Philadelphia: Saunders; 2003. p. 311–47.

22. Perloff JK. Patent ductus arteriosus. In: Perloff JK, editor. Clinical recognition of congenital heart disease. 5th edition. Philadelphia: Saunders; 2003. p. 403–29.

23. Rudolph AM, Scarpelli EM, Golinko RJ, et al. Hemodynamic basis for clinical manifestations of patent ductus arteriosus. Am Heart J 1964;68:447.

24. Murphy PB. The fetal circulation. Continuing education in anaethesia. Crit Care Pain 2005;5:107–12.

25. Rudolph AM. The changes in the circulation after birth. Their importance in congenital heart disease. Circulation 1970;41:343–59.

26. St John Sutton MG, Gewitz MH, Shah B, et al. Quantitative assessment of growth and function of the cardiac chambers in the normal human fetus: a prospective longitudinal echocardiographic study. Circulation 1984;69:645–54.

27. Naito H, Arisawa J, Harada K, et al. Assessment of right ventricular regional contraction and comparison with the left ventricle in normal humans: a cine magnetic resonance study with presaturation myocardial tagging. Br Heart J 1995;74:186–91.

28. Murphy JG, Gersh BJ, McGoon MD, et al. Long-term outcome after surgical repair of isolated atrial septal defect. Follow-up at 27 to 32 years. N Engl J Med 1990;323:1645–50.

29. Konstantinides S, Geibel A, Olschewski M, et al. A comparison of surgical and medical therapy for atrial septal defect in adults. N Engl J Med 1995; 333:469–73.

30. Gatzoulis MA, Freeman MA, Siu SC, et al. Atrial arrhythmia after surgical closure of atrial septal defects in adults. N Engl J Med 1999;340:839–46.

31. Kobayashi J, Yamamoto F, Nakano K, et al. Maze procedure for atrial fibrillation associated with atrial septal defect. Circulation 1998;98(Suppl 2): 399–402.

32. Wagenvoort CA, Neufeld HN, DuShane JW, et al. The pulmonary arterial tree in ventricular septal defect: a quantitative study of anatomic features in fetuses, infants, and children. Circulation 1961;23: 740–8.

33. Wood P. The Eisenmenger syndrome or pulmonary hypertension with reversed central shunt. Br Med J 1958;2:755–62.

34. Perloff JK, Rosove MH, Sietsema KE, et al. Cyanotic congenital heart disease: a multisystem disorder. In: Perloff JK, Child JS, editors. Congenital heart disease in adults. 2nd edition. Philadelphia: W.B. Saunders; 1998. p. 199–226.

35. Niwa K, Perloff JK, Kaplan S, et al. Eisenmenger syndrome in adults: ventricular septal defect, truncus arteriosus, univentricular heart. J Am Coll Cardiol 1999;34:223–32.

36. McElhinney DB, Goldmuntz E. Double-chambered right ventricle. In: Gatzoulis MA, Webb GD, editors. Diagnosis and management of adult congenital heart disease. New York: Churchill Livingstone; 2003. p. 305–11.

37. Thorson AH. Endocardial sclerosis and other heart lesions in the carcinoid disease. Acta Med Scand Suppl 1958;334:99–119.

38. Robiolio PA, Rigolin VH, Wilson JS, et al. Carcinoid heart disease: correlation of high serotonin levels with valvular abnormalities detected by cardiac catheterization and echocardiography. Circulation 1995;92:790–5.

39. Ryan WH, Herbert MA, Dewey TM, et al. The occurrence of postoperative pulmonary homograft stenosis in adult patients undergoing the Ross procedure. J Heart Valve Dis 2006;15:108–13.

40. Fyler DC. Rheumatic fever. In: Keane JK, Lock JE, Fyler DC, editors. Nadas' pediatric cardiology. 2nd edition. Philadelphia: Saunders; 2006. p. 389–90.

41. Connolly HM, Crary JL, McGoon MD, et al. Valvular heart disease associated with fenfluramine-phentermine. N Engl J Med 1997;337:581–8.

42. Perloff JK. Ventricular septal defect with pulmonary stenosis. In: Perloff JK, editor. Clinical recognition of congenital heart disease. 5th edition. Philadelphia: Saunders; 2003. p. 348–82.

43. Nollert G, Fischlein T, Bouterwek DM, et al. Long-term survival in patients with repair of tetralogy of Fallot: 36-year follow-up of 490 survivors of the first year after surgical repair. J Am Coll Cardiol 1997; 30:1374–83.

44. Bouzas B, Kilner PJ, Gatzoulis MA. Pulmonary regurgitation: not a benign lesion. Eur Heart J 2005;26: 433–9.

45. Geva T, Sandweiss BM, Gauvreau K, et al. Factors associated with impaired clinical status in long-term survivors of tetralogy of Fallot repair evaluated by magnetic resonance imaging. J Am Coll Cardiol 2004;43:1068–74.

46. d'Udekem Y, Ovaert C, Grandjean F, et al. Tetralogy of Fallot: transannular and right ventricular patching equally affect late functional status. Circulation 2000;102(Suppl 3):116–22.

47. Pigula FA, Khalil PN, Mayer JE, et al. Repair of tetralogy of Fallot in neonates and young infants. Circulation 1999;100(Suppl 2):157–61.

48. Van Arsdell GS, Maharaj GS, Tom J, et al. What is the optimal age for repair of tetralogy of Fallot? Circulation 2000;102(Suppl 3):123–9.

49. Babu-Narayan SV, Kilner PJ, Li W, et al. Ventricular fibrosis suggested by cardiovascular magnetic resonance in adults with repaired tetralogy of Fallot and its relationship to adverse markers of clinical outcome. Circulation 2006;113:405–13.

50. Chaturvedi RR, Shore DF, Lincoln C, et al. Acute right ventricular restrictive physiology after repair of tetralogy of Fallot: association with myocardial injury and oxidative stress. Circulation 1999;100: 1540–7.

51. Harrild DM, Berul CI, Cecchin F, et al. Pulmonary valve replacement in tetralogy of Fallot: impact on survival and ventricular tachycardia. Circulation 2009;119:445–51.

52. Therrien J, Siu SC, McLaughlin PR, et al. Pulmonary valve replacement in adults late after repair of tetralogy of Fallot: are we operating too late? J Am Coll Cardiol 2000;36:1670–5.

53. Earing MG, Connolly HM, Dearani JA, et al. Long-term follow-up of patients after surgical treatment for isolated pulmonary valve stenosis. Mayo Clin Proc 2005;80:871–6.

54. Rhodes JF, Hijazi ZM, Sommer RJ. Pathophysiology of congenital heart disease in the adult, Part II: simple obstructive lesions. Circulation 2008;117:1228–37.

55. Termignon JL, Leca F, Vouhe PR, et al. "Classic" repair of congenitally corrected transposition and ventricular septal defect. Ann Thorac Surg 1996;62:199–206.

56. Van Son JA, Danielson GK, Huhta JC, et al. Late results of systemic atrioventricular valve replacement in corrected transposition. J Thorac Cardiovasc Surg 1995;109:642–53.

57. Konstantinov IE, Williams WG. Atrial switch and rastelli operation for congenitally corrected transposition with ventricular septal defect and pulmonary stenosis. Op Tech Thorac Cardiovasc Surg 2003;8:160–6.

58. Langley SM, Winlaw DS, Stumper O, et al. Midterm results after restoration of the morphologically left ventricle to the systemic circulation in patients with congenitally corrected transposition of the great arteries. J Thorac Cardiovasc Surg 2003;125: 1229–41.

59. Beghetti M, Galiè N. Eisenmenger Syndrome: a clinical perspective in a new therapeutic era of pulmonary arterial hypertension. J Am Coll Cardiol 2009;53:733–40.

60. Galiè N, Beghetti M, Gatzoulis MA, et al. Bosentan therapy in patients with Eisenmenger syndrome: a multicenter, double-blind, randomized, placebo-controlled study. Circulation 2006;114:48–54.

61. Dimopoulos K, Inuzuka R, Goletto S, et al. Improved survival among patients with Eisenmenger syndrome receiving advanced therapy for pulmonary arterial hypertension. Circulation 2010;121:20–5.

62. Zhang ZN, Jiang X, Zhang R, et al. Oral sildenafil treatment for Eisenmenger syndrome: a prospective, open-label, multicentre study. Heart 2011;22: 1876–81.

63. Mukhopadhyay S, Sharma M, Ramakrishnan S, et al. Phosphodiesterase-5 inhibitor in Eisenmenger syndrome: a preliminary observational study. Circulation 2006;114:1807–18.

Acute Right Ventricular Infarction

James A. Goldstein, MD

KEYWORDS

- Right ventricular ischemia • Right atrial ischemia
- Systolic ventricular interactions • Reperfusion

Based on early experiments of right ventricular (RV) performance, for many years practitioners believed that RV contraction was unimportant in the circulation and, despite loss of RV contraction, pulmonary flow could be generated by a passive gradient from a distended venous system and active right atrial contraction.[1] However, the profound hemodynamic effects of RV systolic dysfunction became evident during the 1970s with the description of severe RV infarction (RVI), resulting in severe right heart failure, clear lungs, and low-output hypotension despite intact global left ventricular (LV) systolic function.[2–4] Nearly 50% of patients with acute ST elevation inferior myocardial infarction (IMI) experience concomitant RVI, which is associated with higher in-hospital morbidity and mortality related to hemodynamic and electrophysiologic complications.[4–6]

Although the magnitude of hemodynamic derangements is related to the extent of RV free wall contraction abnormalities,[6,7] some patients tolerate severe RV systolic dysfunction without hemodynamic compromise, whereas others develop life-threatening low output, emphasizing that additional factors modulate the clinical expression of RVI. Importantly, the term *RV infarction* is to an extent a misnomer, because in most cases acute RV ischemic dysfunction seems to represent viable myocardium, which recovers over time, especially after successful reperfusion and even after prolonged occlusion.[6,8–10]

This article reviews the pathophysiology, hemodynamics, natural history, and management of patients with IMI complicated by RVI. Key areas are highlighted in which advances may impact catheterization and laboratory management of these acutely ill patients, including:

- The relationship between the site of right coronary artery (RCA) occlusion and the presence and magnitude of right heart ischemia and its complications.
- The pathophysiologic mechanisms leading to hemodynamic compromise and their relevance to pharmacologic and mechanical interventions.
- Bradyarrhythmias and tachyarrhythmias complicating management during acute occlusion and reperfusion.
- The concept that *RV infarction* is actually a misnomer, because even severe acute ischemic RV dysfunction is almost always reversible.
- The compensatory mechanisms maintaining hemodynamic performance under conditions of profound RV pump function.
- The benefits of primary catheter-based reperfusion on hemodynamics and clinical outcome, even after prolonged occlusion and in patients with severe shock.

PATTERNS OF CORONARY COMPROMISE RESULTING IN RVI

Significant RVI almost always occurs in association with acute transmural inferior-posterior LV myocardial infarction, and the RCA is always the culprit vessel,[10] typically a proximal occlusion compromising flow to one or more of the major RV branches (**Figs. 1** and **2**). In contrast, distal RCA occlusions or circumflex culprits that spare RV branch perfusion rarely compromise RV performance. Occasionally, isolated RVI may develop from occlusion of a nondominant RCA or selective compromise of RV branches during percutaneous interventions.

Department of Cardiovascular Medicine, Beaumont Health System, 3601 West 13 Mile Road, Royal Oak, MI 48073, USA
E-mail address: JGOLDSTEIN@beaumont.edu

Cardiol Clin 30 (2012) 219–232
doi:10.1016/j.ccl.2012.03.002
0733-8651/12/$ – see front matter © 2012 Published by Elsevier Inc.

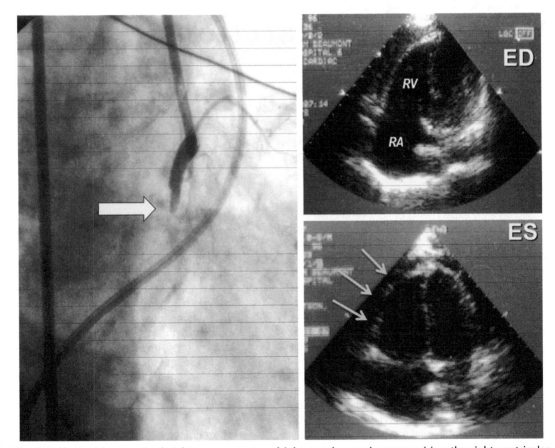

Fig. 1. Patient with a proximal right coronary artery (*right panel, arrow*) compromising the right ventricular branches and resulting in severe RVI, indicated on echocardiogram as severe RV free wall dysfunction and depressed global RV performance at end systole (ES) and marked RV dilation at end diastole (ED).

At necropsy, RVI inscribes a tripartite signature consisting of LV inferior-posterior wall, septal, and posterior RV free wall necrosis contiguous with the septum.[11] However, these autopsy patterns do not reflect most patients who survive acute RVI, because even in the absence of reperfusion of the infarct-related artery, most patients with severe ischemic RV dysfunction manifest spontaneous early hemodynamic improvement and later recovery of RV function.[6–9] In fact, chronic right heart failure attributable to RVI is rare. Thus, the term *RV infarction* is to an extent a misnomer, because in most cases acute RV ischemic dysfunction seems to represent predominantly viable myocardium. These responses are in marked contrast to the effects of ischemia on the LV.[12–14]

RV MECHANICS AND OXYGEN SUPPLY-DEMAND

The right and left ventricles differ markedly in their anatomy, mechanics, loading conditions, and metabolism. Therefore, they have strikingly different oxygen supply and demand characteristics,[15–17] and thus manifest disparate responses to ischemic insults. The LV is a thick-walled pressure pump. In contrast, the pyramidal-shaped RV with its thin crescentic free wall is designed as a volume pump, ejecting into the lower resistance pulmonary circulation. RV systolic pressure and flow are generated by RV free wall shortening and contraction toward the septum from apex to outflow tract.[6,17] The septum is an integral architectural and mechanical component of the RV chamber and, even under physiologic conditions, LV septal contraction contributes to RV performance. The RV has a more favorable oxygen supply-demand profile than the LV. RV oxygen demand is lower owing to lesser myocardial mass, preload, and afterload.[15,16] RV perfusion also is more favorable because of the dual anatomic supply system from left coronary branches. Furthermore, the RV free wall is thinner, develops lower systolic intramyocardial pressure, and experiences less diastolic intracavitary pressure, and lower coronary resistance favors acute collateral development to the RCA.[18]

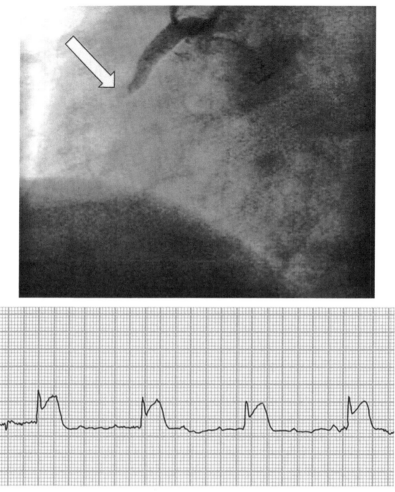

Fig. 2. Patient with proximal right coronary artery occlusion (*arrow*) complicated by third-degree AV block. (*From* Goldstein JA, Lee DT, Pica MC, et al. Patterns of coronary compromise leading to bradyarrhythmias and hypotension in inferior myocardial infarction. Coron Artery Dis 2005;16:267; with permission.)

EFFECTS OF ISCHEMIA ON RV SYSTOLIC AND DIASTOLIC FUNCTION

Proximal RCA occlusion compromises RV free wall perfusion, resulting in RV free wall dyskinesis and depressed global RV performance reflected in the RV waveform by a sluggish, depressed, and systolic waveform (**Figs. 3** and **4**).[7,10,19–23] RV systolic dysfunction diminishes transpulmonary delivery of LV preload, leading to decreased cardiac output despite intact LV contractility. Biventricular diastolic dysfunction contributes to hemodynamic compromise.[19–23] The ischemic RV is stiff and dilated early in diastole, which impedes inflow, leading to rapid diastolic pressure elevation. Acute RV dilatation and elevated diastolic pressure shift the interventricular septum toward the volume-deprived LV, further impairing LV compliance and filling. Abrupt RV dilatation

within the noncompliant pericardium elevates intrapericardial pressure, with the resultant constraint further impairing RV and LV compliance and filling. These effects contribute to the pattern of equalized diastolic pressures and RV "dip-and-plateau" characteristic of RVI.[19–23]

DETERMINANTS OF RV PERFORMANCE IN SEVERE RVI
Importance of Systolic Ventricular Interactions

Despite the absence of RV free wall motion, an active albeit depressed RV systolic waveform is generated through systolic interactions mediated by primary septal contraction and through mechanical displacement of the septum into the RV cavity associated with paradoxic septal motion (see **Fig. 1**).[7,20–23] In the LV, acute ischemia results in regional dyskinesis; these dyssynergic segments

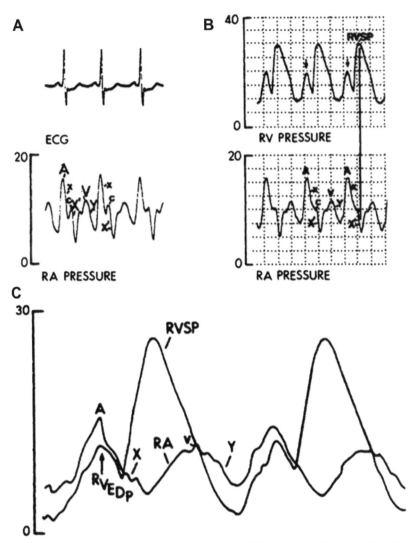

Fig. 3. Hemodynamic recordings from a patient with right atrial (RA) pressure W pattern, timed to electrocardio-gram (ECG) (*A*) and RV pressures (*B* and *C*). Peaks of W are formed by prominent A waves with an associated sharp X systolic descent, followed by a comparatively blunted Y descent. Peak RV systolic pressure (RVSP) is depressed, RV relaxation is prolonged, and a dip and rapid rise occur in RV end-diastolic pressure (RVEPD). (*From* Goldstein JA, Barzilai B, Rosamond TL, et al. Determinants of hemodynamic compromise with severe right ventricular infarc-tion. Circulation 1990;82:359; with permission.)

are stretched in early isovolumic systole by neigh-boring contracting segments through regional intra-ventricular interactions that dissipate the functional work of these neighboring regions.[24] The ischemic dyskinetic RV free wall behaves similarly and must be stretched to the maximal extent of its systolic lengthening through interventricular interactions before providing a stable buttress on which actively contracting segments can generate effective stroke work, thereby imposing a mechanical disadvantage that reduces contributions to cardiac perfor-mance.[20–23] The compensatory contributions of LV septal contraction are emphasized by the

deleterious effects of LV septal dysfunction, which exacerbates hemodynamic compromise associ-ated with RVI.[23] In contrast, inotropic stimulation enhances LV septal contraction and thereby augments RV performance through augmented compensatory systolic interactions.

Compensatory Role of Augmented Right Atrial Contraction

The hemodynamic benefits of augmented atrial contraction to performance of the ischemic LV are well documented.[25] Similarly, augmented right

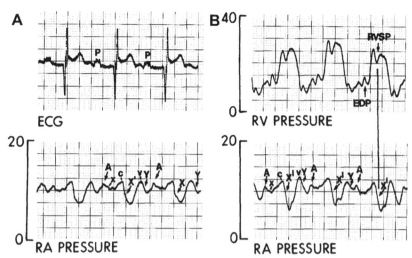

Fig. 4. Right atrial (RA) pressure M pattern timed to electrocardiogram (ECG) (*A*) and RV pressure (*B*). M pattern comprises a depressed A wave, X descent before a small C wave, a prominent X descent, a small V wave, and a blunted Y descent. Peak RV systolic pressure (RVSP) is depressed and bifid (*arrow*), with delayed relaxation and an elevated end-diastolic pressure (EDP) (all pressures are measured in mm Hg). (*From* Goldstein JA, Barzilai B, Rosamond TL, et al. Determinants of hemodynamic compromise with severe right ventricular infarction. Circulation 1990;82:359; with permission.)

atrial (RA) booster pump transport is an important compensatory mechanism that optimizes RV performance and cardiac output.[20–23] When RVI develops from occlusions compromising RV but sparing RA branches, RV diastolic dysfunction imposes increased preload and afterload on the right atrium, resulting in enhanced RA contractility that augments RV filling and performance. This function is reflected in the RA waveform as a "W" pattern characterized by a rapid upstroke and increased peak A wave amplitude, sharp X descent reflecting enhanced atrial relaxation, and blunted Y descent owing to pandiastolic RV dysfunction (see **Fig. 3**).

Deleterious Impact of Right Atrial Ischemia

Conversely, more proximal RCA occlusions compromising atrial and RV branches result in ischemic depression of atrial function, which compromises RV performance and cardiac output.[20–23] RA ischemia manifests hemodynamically as more severely elevated mean RA pressure and inscribes an "M" pattern in the RA waveform characterized by a depressed A wave and X descent and blunted Y descent (see **Fig. 4**). Ischemic atrial involvement is not rare, with autopsy studies documenting atrial infarction in up to 20% of cases of ventricular infarction, with RA involvement five times more common than left.[26,27] Under conditions of acute RV dysfunction, loss of augmented RA transport from ischemic depression of atrial contractility or AV dyssynchrony precipitates more severe

hemodynamic compromise.[20–23] RA dysfunction decreases RV filling, which impairs global RV systolic performance, thereby resulting in further decrements in LV preload and cardiac output. Impaired RA contraction diminishes atrial relaxation; thus, RA ischemia impedes venous return and right heart filling owing to loss of atrial suction associated with atrial relaxation during the X descent.

NATURAL HISTORY OF ISCHEMIC RV DYSFUNCTION

Although RVI may result in profound acute hemodynamic effects, arrhythmias, and higher in-hospital mortality, many patients spontaneously improve within 3 to 10 days regardless of the patency status of the infarct-related artery.[7–9] Furthermore, global RV performance typically recovers, with normalization within 3 to 12 months. Moreover, chronic unilateral right heart failure secondary to RVI is rare.[9] This favorable natural history of RV performance is in marked contrast to the effects of coronary occlusion on segmental and global LV function.[13,14] Observations from experimental animal studies confirm spontaneous recovery of RV function despite chronic RCA occlusion attributable to the more favorable oxygen supply-demand characteristics of the RV in general, and the beneficial effects of collaterals in particular.[28] Similarly, in patients with chronic proximal RCA occlusion, RV function is typically maintained at rest and augments appropriately during stress.[9] The relative resistance of the RV free wall to infarction is undoubtedly attributable to more favorable oxygen supply-demand characteristics. Preinfarction angina seems to reduce the risk of developing RVI, possibly because of preconditioning.[18]

EFFECTS OF REPERFUSION ON ISCHEMIC RV DYSFUNCTION

Although RV function may recover despite persistent RCA occlusion, acute RV ischemia contributes to early morbidity and mortality.[4–6] Furthermore, spontaneous recovery of RV contractile function and hemodynamics may be slow. The beneficial effects of successful reperfusion in patients with predominant LV infarction are well documented.[12–14] Observations in experimental animals[29] and in humans[30] now show the beneficial effects of reperfusion on recovery of RV performance. In patients,[7] successful mechanical reperfusion of the RCA, including the major RV branches, leads to immediate improvement in and later complete recovery of RVFW function and global RV performance (**Fig. 5**). Reperfusion-mediated recovery of RV performance

is associated with excellent clinical outcome (**Fig. 6**). In contrast, failure to restore flow to the major RV branches was associated with lack of recovery of RV performance and refractory hemodynamic compromise, leading to high in-hospital mortality, even if flow was restored in the main RCA. Findings now also show that successful mechanical reperfusion leads to superior late survival of patients with shock from predominant RVI versus those with LV shock.[31]

Although evidence suggests that patients with IMI benefit from timely thrombolytic reperfusion, the specific short-term and long-term responses of those with RVI have not been adequately evaluated. Some thrombolytic studies suggested that RV function improves only in patients in whom RCA patency is achieved,[32–35] whereas others report little benefit.[35,36] More recent prospective reports show that successful thrombolysis imparts survival benefit in those with RV involvement and that failure to restore infarct-related artery patency is associated with persistent RV dysfunction and increased mortality.[36] Unfortunately, patients with RVI seem to be particularly resistant to fibrinolytic recanalization, owing to proximal RCA occlusion with extensive clot burden which,

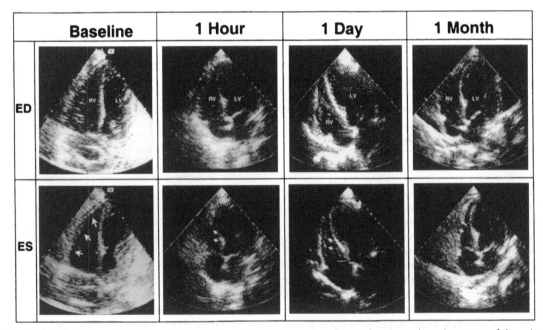

Fig. 5. Echocardiographic images from a patient with acute IMI and RV ischemia undergoing successful angioplasty. End-diastolic and end-systolic images obtained at baseline show severe RV dilatation with reduced LV diastolic size. At ES, there was RVFW dyskinesis (*arrows*), intact LV function and compensatory paradoxical septal motion. One hour after angioplasty, there was striking recovery of RVFW contraction (*arrows*), resulting in marked improvement in global RV performance and markedly increased RV size and LV preload. At one day, there was further improvement in RV function (*arrows*), which at one month was normal. RV denotes right ventricle while LV denotes left ventricle. (*From* Bowers TR, O'Neill WW, Grines C, et al. Effect of reperfusion on biventricular function and survival after right ventricular infarction. N Eng J Med 1998;338:933; with permission.)

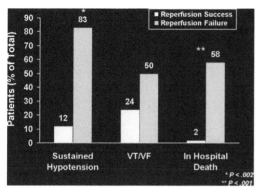

Fig. 6. Bar graphs demonstrating benefits of successful reperfusion versus reperfusion failure with respect to reduced arrhythmias, sustained hypotension and in-hospital survival. (*From* Bowers TR, O'Neill WW, Grines C, et al. Effect of reperfusion on biventricular function and survival after right ventricular infarction. N Eng J Med 1998;338:933; with permission.)

together with impaired coronary delivery of fibrinolytic agents, is attributable to hypotension.[36] A higher incidence of reocclusion also seems to occur after thrombolysis of the RCA.

RVI is important to consider separately in the elderly. Early reports suggested that elderly patients with RVI experience 50% in-hospital mortality and that hemodynamic compromise in these cases is irreversible. However, recent studies document that most patients with RVI who undergo successful mechanical reperfusion survive, including those with hemodynamic compromise.[37]

RHYTHM DISORDERS AND REFLEXES ASSOCIATED WITH RVI
Bradyarrhythmias and Hypotension

High-grade atrioventricular (AV) block and bradycardia-hypotension without AV block commonly complicate IMI and have been attributed predominantly to the effects of AV nodal ischemia and cardioinhibitory (Bezold-Jarisch) reflexes arising from stimulation of vagal afferents in the ischemic LV inferoposterior wall.[38–42] Patients with acute RVI are at increased risk for both high-grade AV block and bradycardia-hypotension without AV block.[4,42] Recent findings now document that during acute coronary occlusion, bradycardia-hypotension and AV block are far more common in patients with proximal RCA lesions (see **Fig. 2**) inducing RV and LV inferior-posterior ischemia, compared with more distal occlusions compromising LV perfusion but sparing the RV branches.[42] These observations suggest that the ischemic right heart may elicit cardioinhibitory-vasodilator reflexes. In patients

with IMI, whose rhythm and blood pressure were stable during occlusion, similar bradycardic hypotensive reflexes may be elicited during reperfusion[42,43] and also seem to be more common with proximal lesions (**Fig. 7**).

Ventricular Arrhythmias

Patients with RVI are prone to ventricular tachyarrhythmias,[4,44] which should not be unexpected given that the ischemic RV is often massively dilated.[44] Autonomic denervation in the periinfarct area may also play a role.[45] In patients with RVI, ventricular tachycardia (VT)/ventricular fibrillation (VF) may develop in a trimodal pattern, either during acute occlusion, abruptly with reperfusion, or later.[44] However, successful mechanical reperfusion dramatically reduces the incidence of malignant ventricular arrhythmias,[7,44] presumably through improvement in RV function, which lessens late VT/VF. Occasionally, RVI may be complicated by recurrent malignant arrhythmias and, in some cases, intractable "electrical storm" (**Fig. 8**), possibly because of sustained severe RV dilatation.[44]

MECHANICAL COMPLICATIONS ASSOCIATED WITH RVI

Patients with acute RVI may experience additional mechanical complications of acute infarction that may compound hemodynamic compromise and confound the clinical hemodynamic picture. Ventricular septal rupture is a particularly disastrous complication, adding substantial overload stress to the isochemically dysfunctional RV, precipitating pulmonary edema, elevating pulmonary pressures and resistance, and exacerbating low output.[46] Surgical repair is imperative but may be technically difficult owing to extensive necrosis involving the LV inferior-posterior free wall, septum, and apex. Catheter closure of these defects may be possible. Severe right heart dilatation and diastolic pressure elevation associated with RVI may stretch open a patent foramen ovale, precipitating acute right-to-left shunting manifest as systemic hypoxemia or paradoxic emboli.[47] Most patent foramen ovale complications abate after successful mechanical reperfusions, because right heart pressures diminish with recovery of RV performance; rarely, some may require percutaneous closure.[48] Severe tricuspid regurgitation may also complicate RVI, developing as a result of primary papillary muscle ischemic dysfunction or rupture and secondary functional regurgitation attributable to severe RV and tricuspid valve annular dilatation.[49]

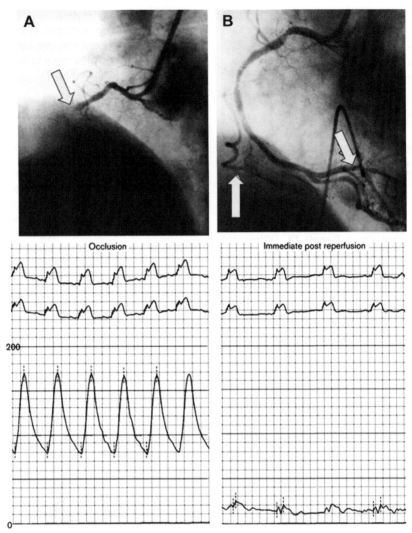

Fig. 7. Patient with a proximal right coronary artery (*left panel, arrow*) compromising the RV branches (*right panel, solid arrow*) as well as the LV and atrioventricular nodal branches (*right panel, open arrow*), who developed profound repefrusion-induced bradycardia-hypotension. Sinus rhythm with normal blood pressure was seen during occlusion. Reperfusion through primary percutaneous transluminal coronary angioplasty resulted in abrupt but transient sinus bradycardia with profound hypotension. PCI, percutaneous coronary intervention. (*From* Goldstein JA, Lee DT, Pica MC, et al. Patterns of coronary compromise leading to bradyarrhythmias and hypotension in inferior myocardial infarction. Coron Artery Dis 2005;16:265–74; with permission.)

CLINICAL PRESENTATIONS AND EVALUATION

RVI is often silent, with only 25% of patients developing clinically evident hemodynamic manifestations.[6] Patients with severe RVI but preserved global LV function may be hemodynamically compensated, manifest by elevated jugular venous pressure but clear lungs, normal systemic arterial pressure, and intact perfusion. When RVI leads to more severe hemodynamic compromise, systemic hypotension and hypoperfusion result. Patients with IMI may initially present without evidence of hemodynamic compromise but subsequently develop hypotension precipitated by preload reduction attributable to nitroglycerin[50] or associated with bradyarrhythmias.[42] When RVI develops in the setting of global LV dysfunction, the picture may be dominated by low output and pulmonary congestion, with right heart failure.

NONINVASIVE AND HEMODYNAMIC EVALUATION

Although ST segment elevation and loss of R wave in the right-sided electrocardiogram leads (V_{3R} and V_{4R}) are sensitive indicators of the presence of RVI,[51,52] they are not predictive of the magnitude of RV dysfunction nor its hemodynamic

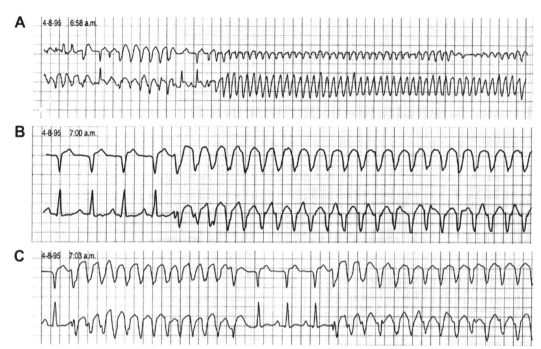

Fig. 8. Electrical storm developing 36 hours after reperfusion. Shown are rhythm strips from 3 of the 5 episodes of VFL or VT that occurred over a 75-minute span. All episodes were successfully terminated with antiarrhythmic agents and defibrillation. The patient died on hospital day 48 from refractory VF. (*From* Ricci JM, Dukkipati SR, Pica MC, et al. Malignant ventricular arrhythmias in patients with acute right ventricular infarction undergoing mechanical reperfusion. Am J Cardiol 2009;104:1678–83.)

impact. Echocardiography is the most effective tool for delineating the presence and severity of RV dilatation and depression of global RV performance.[6] Echocardiography also delineates the extent of reversed septal curvature that confirms the presence of significant adverse diastolic interactions, the degree of paradoxic septal motion indicative of compensatory systolic interactions, and the presence of severe RA enlargement, which may indicate concomitant ischemic RA dysfunction and/or tricuspid regurgitation. Recent observations from cardiac MRI studies suggest that the extent of acute RV dysfunction and RV free wall myonecrosis (indicated by late gadolinium enhancement and obstruction) are independent predictors of long-term outcome.[53] The extent of LV infarction was also a key predictor of outcome. Because global RV performance is dependent on LV septal function when the RV free wall is impaired, it is not surprising that more extensive biventricular infarction and systolic dysfunction would exert more profound acute hemodynamic compromise and portend adverse prognosis.

Invasive hemodynamic assessment of the extent and severity of right heart ischemic involvement has been extensively discussed.

DIFFERENTIAL DIAGNOSIS OF RVI

Important clinical entities to consider in patients who present with acute low output hypotension, clear lungs, and disproportionate right heart failure include cardiac tamponade, acute pulmonary embolism, severe pulmonary hypertension, right heart mass obstruction, and acute severe tricuspid regurgitation. Entities such as constrictive pericarditis or restrictive cardiomyopathy present a similar picture but are not acute processes (**Box 1**). The general clinical presentation of chest pain with acute IMI, together with echocardiographic documentation of RV dilatation and dysfunction, effectively excludes tamponade, constriction, and restriction. Acute massive pulmonary embolism may also mimic severe RVI and, because the unprepared RV cannot acutely generate elevated RV systolic pressures (>50–55 mm Hg), severe pulmonary hypertension may be absent. In these cases, absence of inferior LV myocardial infarction on electrocardiogram and echocardiogram indicate embolism, which is easily confirmed with CT or invasive angiography. Severe pulmonary hypertension with RV decompensation may mimic severe RVI, but delineation of markedly elevated PA systolic pressures on Doppler or invasive hemodynamic monitoring excludes RVI, in which RV pressure generation is depressed. Acute primary tricuspid regurgitation should be evident on echocardiography, typically caused by infective endocarditis with obvious vegetations.

THERAPY

Therapeutic options for the management of right heart ischemia (**Box 2**) follow directly from the pathophysiology discussed. Treatment modalities include (1) restoration of physiologic rhythm, (2) optimization of ventricular preload, (3) optimization of oxygen supply and demand, (4) parenteral inotropic support for persistent hemodynamic compromise, (5) reperfusion, and (6) mechanical support with intraaortic balloon counterpulsation and RV assist devices.

Physiologic Rhythm

Patients with RVI are particularly prone to the adverse effects of bradyarrhythmias. The depressed ischemic RV has a relatively fixed stroke

volume, as does the preload-deprived LV. Therefore, biventricular output is exquisitely heart rate–dependent, and bradycardia even in the absence of AV dyssynchrony may be deleterious to patients with RVI. For similar reasons, chronotropic competence is critical in patients with RVI. However, these patients not only are notoriously prone to reflex-mediated frank bradycardia but also often manifest a relative inability to increase the sinus rate in response to low output, owing to excess vagal tone, ischemia, or pharmacologic agents. Given that the ischemic RV is dependent on atrial transport, the loss of RA contraction from AV dyssynchrony further exacerbates difficulties with RV filling and contributes to hemodynamic compromise.[6,20,21] Although atropine may restore physiologic rhythm in some patients, temporary pacing is often required. Although ventricular pacing alone may suffice, especially if the bradyarrhythmias are intermittent, some patients require AV sequential pacing.[54] However, transvenous pacing can be difficult because of issues with ventricular sensing, presumably related to diminished generation of endomyocardial potentials in the ischemic RV. Manipulating catheters within the dilated ischemic RV may also induce ventricular arrhythmias.[44] Intravenous aminophylline may restore sinus rhythm in some patients with atropine-resistant AV block, a response likely reflecting reversal of ischemia-induced adenosine elaboration.[55,56]

Optimization of Preload

In patients with RVI, the dilated noncompliant RV is exquisitely preload-dependent, as is the LV, which is stiff but preload-deprived. Therefore, any factor that reduces ventricular preload tends to be detrimental. Accordingly, vasodilators and diuretics are contraindicated. Although experimental animal studies of RVI show hemodynamic benefit from volume loading,[57] clinical studies have reported variable responses to volume challenge.[58–60] These conflicting results may reflect a spectrum of initial volume status in patients with acute RVI, with patients who are volume-depleted experiencing benefit and those who are more volume-replete manifesting a flat response to fluid resuscitation. Nevertheless, an initial volume challenge is appropriate for patients manifesting low output without pulmonary congestion, particularly if the estimated central venous pressure is less than 15 mm Hg. For those who experience no response to an initial trail of fluids, determination of filling pressures and subsequent hemodynamically monitored volume challenge may be appropriate. Caution should be exercised to avoid excessive volume administration above and beyond that documented to augment output, because the right heart chambers may operate on a descending limb of the Starling curve, resulting in further depression of RV pump performance and inducing severe systemic venous congestion. Abnormalities of volume retention and impaired diuresis may be related partly to impaired responses of the atrial natriuretic factor.[61]

Anti-Ischemic Therapies

Treatment of RVI should focus on optimizing oxygen supply-demand to optimize recovery of both LV and RV function and LV function. However, most anti-ischemic agents exert hemodynamic effects, which may be deleterious in patients with RVI. Specially, β-blockers and some calcium channel blockers may reduce heart rate and depress conduction, thereby increasing the risk of bradyarrhythmias and heart block in these chrono-tropically dependent patients. The vasodilator pro-perties of nitrates and calcium channel blockers may precipitate hypotension. In general, these drugs should be avoided in patients with RVI.

Reperfusion Therapy

The beneficial effects of successful reperfusion on RV function and clinical outcome, and the demon-strated efficacy and advantages of primary an-gioplasty versus thrombolysis in patients with acute right heart ischemic dysfunction, have been discussed.

Inotropic Stimulation

Parenteral inotropic support is usually effective in stabilizing hemodynamically compromised pa-tients not fully responsive to volume resuscitation and restoration of physiologic rhythm.[7,23,58] The mechanisms through which inotropic stimulation improve low output and hypotension in patients with acute RVI have not been well studied. How-ever, experimental animal investigations suggest that inotropic stimulation enhances RV perfor-mance through increasing LV septal contraction, which thereby augments septal-mediated systolic ventricular interactions.[23] Although an inotropic agent, such as dobutamine, that has the least deleterious effects on afterload, oxygen consump-tion, and arrhythmias is the preferred initial drug, patients with severe hypotension may require agents with pressor effects (such as dopamine) for prompt restoration of adequate coronary perfu-sion pressure. The inodilator agents, such as milri-none, have not been studied in patients with RVI, but their vasodilator properties could exacerbate hypotension.

Mechanical Assist Devices

Intraaortic balloon pumping may be beneficial in patients with RVI and refractory low output and hypotension. Although little research is available to shed light on the mechanisms through which it exerts salutary effects, balloon assist likely does not directly improve RV performance, but stabi-lizes blood pressure and thereby improves perfu-sion pressure throughout the coronary tree in severely hypotensive patients. Because RV my-ocardial blood flow is dependent on perfusion pressure, balloon pumping may therefore also improve RV perfusion and thereby benefit RV func-tion, particularly if the RCA has been recanalized or if there is collateral supply to an occluded vessel. Intraaortic balloon pumping may also potentially improve LV performance in patients with hypotension and depressed LV function. Because performance of the dysfunctional RV is largely dependent on LV septal contraction, RV performance may also benefit. Recent reports suggest that percutaneous RV assist devices can improve hemodynamics in patients with refractory life-threatening low output, thereby providing the reperfused RV a bridge to recovery.[62,63]

SUMMARY

Acute RCA occlusion proximal to the RV branches results in RV free wall dysfunction. The ischemic dyskinetic RV free wall exerts mechanically disad-vantageous effects on biventricular performance. Depressed RV systolic function leads to a dimin-ished transpulmonary delivery of LV preload, re-sulting in reduced cardiac output. The ischemic RV is stiff, dilated, and volume-dependent, result-ing in pandiastolic RV dysfunction and septally mediated alterations in LV compliance, exacer-bated by elevated intrapericardial pressure. Under these conditions, RV pressure generation and output are dependent on LV septal contraction and paradoxic septal motion. Culprit lesions distal to the RA branches augment RA contractility and enhance RV filling and performance. Bradyar-rhythmias limit the output generated by the rate-dependent ventricles. Ventricular arrhythmias are common, but do not impact short-term outcomes if mechanical reperfusion is prompt. Patients with RVI and hemodynamic instability often respond to volume resuscitation and restoration of phy-siologic rhythm. Vasodilators and diuretics should generally be avoided. In some patients, parenteral inotropes are required. The RV is resistant to infarction and usually recovers even after pro-longed occlusion. However, prompt reperfusion enhances recovery of RV performance and improves the clinical course and survival of patients with ischemic RV dysfunction.

REFERENCES

1. Starr I, Jeffers WA, Meade RH. The absence of conspicuous increments of venous pressure after severe damage to the right ventricle of the dog, with a discussion of the relation between clinical congestive failure and heart disease. Am Heart J 1943;26:291–301.
2. Cohn JN, Guiha NH, Broder MI, et al. Right ventricular infarction. Clinical and hemodynamic features. Am J Cardiol 1974;33:209–14.
3. Lorell B, Leinbach RC, Pohost GM, et al. Right ventricular infarction: clinical diagnosis and differentiation from cardiac tamponade and pericardial constriction. Am J Cardiol 1979;43:465–71.
4. Zehender M, Kasper W, Kauder E, et al. Right ventricular infarction as an independent predictor of prognosis after acute inferior myocardial infarction. N Engl J Med 1993;328:981–8.
5. Jacobs AK, Leopold JA, Bates E, et al. Cardiogenic shock caused by right ventricular infarction: a report from the SHOCK registry. J Am Coll Cardiol 2003;41:1273–9.
6. Goldstein JA. State of the art review: pathophysiology and management of right heart ischemia. J Am Coll Cardiol 2002;40:841–53.
7. Bowers TR, O'Neill WW, Grines C, et al. Effect of reperfusion on biventricular function and survival after right ventricular infarction. N Engl J Med 1998;338:933–40.
8. Dell'Italia LJ, Lembo NJ, Starling MR, et al. Hemodynamically important right ventricular infarction: follow-up evaluation of right ventricular systolic function at rest and during exercise with radionuclide ventriculography and respiratory gas exchange. Circulation 1987;75:996–1003.
9. Lim ST, Marcovitz P, Pica M, et al. Right ventricular performance at rest and during stress with chronic proximal occlusion of the right coronary artery. Am J Cardiol 2003;92:1203–6.
10. Bowers TR, O'Neill WW, Pica M, et al. Patterns of coronary compromise resulting in acute right ventricular ischemic dysfunction. Circulation 2002;106(9):1104–9.
11. Andersen HR, Falk E, Nielsen D. Right ventricular infarction: frequency, size and topography in coronary heart disease: a prospective study compromising 107 consecutive autopsies from a coronary care unit. J Am Coll Cardiol 1987;10:1223–32.
12. Bush LR, Buja LM, Samowitz W, et al. Recovery of left ventricular segmental function after long-term reperfusion following temporary coronary occlusion in conscious dogs. Circ Res 1983;3:248–63.
13. O'Neill WW, Timmis GC, Bourdillon PD, et al. A prospective randomized clinical trial of intracoronary streptokinase versus coronary angioplasty for acute myocardial infarction. N Engl J Med 1986;314:812–8.
14. Bates ER, Califf RM, Stack RS, et al. Thrombolysis and angioplasty in myocardial infarction (TAMI-1) trial: influence of infarct location on arterial patency, left ventricular function and mortality. J Am Coll Cardiol 1989;1:12–8.
15. Kusachi S, Nishiyama O, Yasuhara K, et al. Right and left ventricular oxygen metabolism in open-chest dogs. Am J Physiol 1982;243:H761–6.
16. Ohzono K, Koyanagi S, Urabe Y, et al. Transmural distribution of myocardial infarction: difference between the right and left ventricles in a canine model. Circ Res 1986;59:63–73.
17. Santamore WP, Lynch PR, Heckman JL, et al. Left ventricular effects on right ventricular developed pressure. J Appl Physiol 1976;41:925–30.
18. Shiraki H, Yoshikawa U, Anzai T, et al. Association between preinfarction angina and a lower risk of right ventricular infarction. N Engl J Med 1998;338:941–7.
19. Goldstein JA, Vlahakes GJ, Verrier ED, et al. The role of right ventricular systolic dysfunction and elevated intrapericardial pressure in the genesis of low output in experimental right ventricular infarction. Circulation 1982;65:513–22.
20. Goldstein JA, Barzilai B, Rosamond TL, et al. Determinants of hemodynamic compromise with severe right ventricular infarction. Circulation 1990;82:259.
21. Goldstein JA, Harada A, Yagi Y, et al. Hemodynamic importance of systolic ventricular interaction augmented right atrial contractility and atrioventricular synchrony in acute right ventricular dysfunction. J Am Coll Cardiol 1990;16:181–9.
22. Goldstein JA, Tweddell JS, Barzilai B, et al. Right atrial ischemia exacerbates hemodynamic compromise associated with experimental right ventricular dysfunction. J Am Coll Cardiol 1991;18:1564–72.
23. Goldstein JA, Tweddell JS, Barzilai B, et al. Importance of left ventricular function and systolic interaction to right ventricular performance during acute right heart ischemia. J Am Coll Cardiol 1992;19:704–11.
24. Akaishi M, Weintraum WS, Schneider RM, et al. Analysis of systolic bulging: mechanical characteristics of acutely ischemic myocardium in the conscious dog. Circ Res 1986;8:209–17.
25. Rahimtoola SH, Ehsani A, Sinno MZ, et al. Left atrial transport function in myocardial infarction. Am J Med 1975;9:686–94.
26. Cushing EH, Feil HS, Stanton EJ, et al. Infarction of the cardiac auricles (atria): clinical, pathological, and experimental studies. Br Heart J 1942;4:17–34.
27. Lasar EJ, Goldberger JH, Peled H, et al. Atrial infarction: diagnosis and management. Am Heart J 1988;6:1058–63.

28. Laster SB, Shelton TJ, Barzilai B, et al. Determinants of the recovery of right ventricular performance following experimental chronic right coronary artery occlusion. Circulation 1993;88:696–708.

29. Laster SB, Ohnishi Y, Saffitz JE, et al. Effects of re-perfusion on ischemic right ventricular dysfunction: disparate mechanisms of benefit related to duration of ischemia. Circulation 1994;90:1398–409.

30. Kinn JW, Ajluni SC, Samyn JG, et al. Rapid hemodynamic improvement after reperfusion during right ventricular infarction. J Am Coll Cardiol 1995;26: 1230–4.

31. Brodie BR, Stuckey TD, Hansen C, et al. Comparison of late survival in patients with cardiogenic shock due to right ventricular infarction versus left ventricular pump failure following primary percutaneous coronary intervention for ST-elevation acute myocardial infarction. Am J Cardiol 2007; 99:431–5.

32. Schuler G, Hofmann M, Schwarz F, et al. Effect of successful thrombolytic therapy on right ventricular function in acute inferior wall myocardial infarction. Am J Cardiol 1984;54:951–7.

33. Braat SH, Ramentol M, Halders S, et al. Reperfusion with streptokinase of an occluded right coronary artery: effects on early and late right ventricular ejection fraction. Am Heart J 1987;113:257–60.

34. Roth A, Miller HI, Kaluski E, et al. Early thrombolytic therapy does not enhance the recovery of the right ventricle in patients with acute inferior myocardial infarction and predominant right ventricular involvement. Cardiology 1990;77:40–9.

35. Giannitsis E, Potratz J, Wiegand U, et al. Impact of early accelerated dose tissue plasminogen activator on in-hospital patency of the infarcted vessel in patients with acute right ventricular infarction. Heart 1997;77:512–6.

36. Zeymer U, Neuhaus KL, Wegscheider K, et al. Effects of thrombolytic therapy in acute inferior myocardial infarction with or without right ventricular involvement. J Am Coll Cardiol 1998;32:876–81.

37. Hanzel G, Merhi WM, O'Neill WW, et al. Impact of mechanical reperfusion on clinical outcome in elderly patients with right ventricular infarction. Coron Artery Dis 2006;17:517–21.

38. Adgey AA, Geddes JS, Mulholland C, et al. Incidence, significance, and management of early bradyarrhythmia complicating acute myocardial infarction. Lancet 1968;2(7578):1097–101.

39. Tans A, Lie K, Durrer D. Clinical setting and prognostic significance of high degree atrioventricular block in acute inferior myocardial infarction: a study of 144 patients. Am Heart J 1980;99:4–8.

40. Wei JY, Markis JE, Malagold M, et al. Cardiovascular reflexes stimulated by reperfusion of ischemic myocardium in acute myocardial infarction. Circulation 1983;67:796–801.

41. Mavric Z, Zaputovic L, Matana A, et al. Prognostic significance of complete atrioventricular block in patients with acute inferior myocardial infarction with and without right ventricular involvement. Am Heart J 1990;19:823–8.

42. Goldstein JA, Lee DT, Pica MC, et al. Patterns of coronary compromise leading to bradyarrhythmias and hypotension in inferior myocardial infarction. Coron Artery Dis 2005;16:265–74.

43. Gacioch GM, Topol EJ. Sudden paradoxic clinical deterioration during angioplasty of the occluded right coronary artery in acute myocardial infarction. J Am Coll Cardiol 1989;14:1202–9.

44. Ricci JM, Dukkipati SR, Pica MC, et al. Malignant ventricular arrhythmias in patients with acute right ventricular infarction undergoing mechanical reperfusion. Am J Cardiol 2009;104:1678–83.

45. Elvan A, Zipes D. Right ventricular infarction causes heterogeneous autonomic denervation of the viable peri-infarct area. Circulation 1998;97:484–92.

46. Moore CA, Nygaard TW, Kaiser DL, et al. Postinfarction ventricular septal rupture: the importance of location of infarction and right ventricular function in determining survival. Circulation 1986;74:45–55.

47. Laham RJ, Ho KK, Douglas PS, et al. Right ventricular infarction complicated by acute right-to-left shunting. Am J Cardiol 1994;74:824–6.

48. Gudipati CV, Nagelhout DA, Serota H, et al. Transesophageal echocardiographic guidance for balloon catheter occlusion of patent foramen ovale complicating right ventricular infarction. Am Heart J 1991; 121(3Pt1):919–22.

49. Korr KS, Levinson H, Bough E, et al. Tricuspid valve replacement for cardiogenic shock after acute right ventricular infarction. JAMA 1980;244:1958–60.

50. Ferguson JJ, Diver DJ, Boldt M, et al. Significance of nitroglycerin-induced hypotension with inferior wall acute myocardial infarction. Am J Cardiol 1989;64: 311–4.

51. Braat SH, Brugada P, deZwaan C, et al. Value of electrocardiogram in diagnosing right ventricular involvement in patients with acute inferior wall myocardial infarction. Br Heart J 1983;49:368–72.

52. Klein HO, Tordjman T, Ninio R, et al. The early recognition of right ventricular infarction: diagnostic accuracy of the electrocardiographic V_4R lead. Circulation 1983;67:558–65.

53. Miszalski-Jamka T, Klimeczek P, Tomala M, et al. Extent of RV dysfunction and myocardial infarction assessed by CMR are independent outcome predictors early after STEMI treated with primary angioplasty. JACC Cardiovasc Imaging 2010;3:1237–46.

54. Topol EJ, Goldschlager N, Ports TA, et al. Hemodynamic benefit of atrial pacing in right ventricular myocardial infarction. Ann Intern Med 1982;6:594–7.

55. Wesley RC, Lerman BB, DiMarco JP, et al. Mechanism of atropine-resistant atrioventricular block

during inferior myocardial infarction: possible role of adenosine. J Am Coll Cardiol 1986;8:1232–4.

56. Goodfellow J, Walker PR. Reversal of atropine-resistant atrioventricular block with intravenous aminophylline in the early phase of inferior wall acute myocardial infarction following treatment with streptokinase. Eur Heart J 1995;16:862–5.

57. Goldstein JA, Vlahakes GJ, Verrier ED, et al. Volume loading improves low cardiac output in experimental right ventricular infarction. J Am Coll Cardiol 1983;2:270–8.

58. Dell'Italia LJ, Starling MR, Blumhardt R, et al. Comparative effects of volume loading, dobutamine, and nitroprusside in patients with predominant right ventricular infarction. Circulation 1985;72(6):1327–35.

59. Siniorakis EE, Nikolaou NI, Sarantopoulos CD, et al. Volume loading in predominant right ventricular infarction: bedside hemodynamics using rapid response thermistors. Eur Heart J 1994;15:1340–7.

60. Ferrario M, Poli A, Previtali M, et al. Hemodynamics of volume loading compared with Dobutamine in severe right ventricular infarction. Am J Cardiol 1994;74:329–33.

61. Robalino BD, Petrella RW, Jubran FY, et al. Atrial Natriuretic factor in patients with right ventricular infarction. J Am Coll Cardiol 1990;15:546–53.

62. Giesler GM, Gomez JS, Letsou G, et al. Initial report of percutaneous right ventricular assist for right ventricular shock secondary to right ventricular infarction. Catheter Cardiovasc Interv 2006;68:263–6.

63. Atiemo AD, Conte JV, Heldman AW. Resuscitation and recovery from acute right ventricular failure using a percutaneous right ventricular assist device. Catheter Cardiovasc Interv 2006;66:78–82.

Right Ventricular Responses to Massive and Submassive Pulmonary Embolism

Christian Castillo, MD[a], Victor F. Tapson, MD[b],*

KEYWORDS

- Right ventricular dysfunction • Right ventricular failure
- Pulmonary embolism • Massive pulmonary embolism
- Submassive pulmonary embolism
- Venous thromboembolism

CLINICAL CASE

A 67-year-old man with a history of hypertension presented to the emergency room with 3 days of dyspnea. He denied leg swelling or pain, chest pain, palpitations, hemoptysis, lightheadedness, or syncope. He also denied any known risk factors for venous thromboembolism (VTE), except for his age. Physical examination revealed an anxious man who easily became dyspneic with minimal exertion. He was afebrile; his heart rate was 88 beats/min, blood pressure 130/92 mm Hg, and respiratory rate 21 breaths/min. The patient was found to be hypoxemic, with an oxygen saturation of 87% on room air. There was no obvious neck vein elevation, audible murmurs, loud P2, or right ventricular (RV) lift. Laboratory findings were notable for the following: (1) D-dimer level that was 10 times the upper limit of normal; (2) negative cardiac troponin level; and (3) pro-brain natriuretic peptide (BNP) level that was high at 1842 pg/mL (reference range, <600 pg/mL). Arterial blood gas analysis revealed a pH of 7.41, P_{CO2} of 32 mm Hg, and P_{O2} of 55 mm Hg on room air. The electrocardiogram did not show a right heart strain pattern. He was placed on 2 L/min of supplemental oxygen, and treatment

dose subcutaneous enoxaparin was initiated. A contrast-enhanced chest computed tomographic angiogram (CTA) demonstrated extensive bilateral pulmonary embolism (PE), involving the right upper, right lower, and left upper lobe segmental and subsegmental pulmonary arteries. Transthoracic echocardiography revealed a moderately enlarged, hypokinetic right ventricle. The patient was admitted to the inpatient hospital ward and discussions regarding the use of thrombolytic therapy immediately ensued.

EPIDEMIOLOGY

Every year, there are as many as 300,000 deaths in the United States from acute PE.[1,2] Unfortunately, the diagnosis is often not made until autopsy.[3,4] The case fatality rate for PE in the first 3 months after diagnosis has been reported to be about 15% to 18%, exceeding the mortality rate for acute myocardial infarction.[5,6] In fact, a prior study of PE demonstrated that sudden death was the initial clinical manifestation in nearly 25% of patients.[7] Acute PE survivors may have sequelae that affect their quality of life, such as chronic thromboembolic pulmonary hypertension or

Dr Castillo has nothing to disclose. Dr Tapson has consulted with companies active in the field of venous thromboembolism, including sanofi Aventis, Bayer, Johnson & Johnson, EKOS, Pfizer, and Boehringer Ingelheim.

[a] Division of Pulmonary and Critical Care Medicine, Duke University Medical Center, Box 2634 DUMC, Durham, NC 27710, USA; [b] Division of Pulmonary, Allergy and Critical Care Medicine, Pulmonary Vascular Disease Center, Duke University Medical Center, Room 128, Hanes House, Durham, NC 27710, USA
* Corresponding author.
E-mail address: tapso001@mc.duke.edu

cardiology.theclinics.com

chronic leg pain and swelling (postthrombotic syndrome).

RISK FACTORS

Certain risk factors increase the likelihood of VTE, including a previous history of VTE. Trauma, major surgery (particularly hip and knee replacement and hip fracture), cancer, and hospitalization for acute medical illnesses (such as pneumonia and congestive heart failure)[8] confer significant risks for thromboembolism. Immobility or markedly reduced mobility also imparts an increased risk. Prolonged air[9] or ground travel appears to increase the risk for VTE, as do advanced age, obesity, and pregnancy.

Hereditary or acquired factors that may lead to a hypercoagulable state and thus increase the risk of thromboembolic events include the following: antithrombin deficiency, protein C deficiency, protein S deficiency, the factor V Leiden mutation resulting in activated protein C resistance, the prothrombin gene 20210 mutation, and the presence of antiphospholipid antibodies. Suspicion and consideration for evaluation of these thrombophilias should arise when (1) there are no apparent risk factors for VTE at all, (2) VTE occurs in young patients or in unusual locations (eg, renal vein thrombosis, cerebral sinus thrombosis), (3) unexplained recurrences develop, (4) there are multiple family members who have had VTE, or (5) recurrent spontaneous abortions occur.[5]

CLASSIFICATIONS OF ACUTE PE

Small to moderate PE commonly occur and are characterized by normotensive patients with preserved RV function.[5] These patients appear clinically well and have an excellent prognosis with therapeutic anticoagulation alone.[5]

Massive PE is a life-threatening condition. The criteria that define massive PE include cardiogenic shock and systemic arterial hypotension. Shock leads to tissue hypoperfusion, hypoxia, and ultimately, multi-organ failure.[10] The emboli are usually bilateral and widespread, typically involving a significant amount of the pulmonary arterial vasculature (main and/or lobar pulmonary arteries); less extensive emboli may be seen when there is underlying cardiopulmonary disease limiting a patient's reserve.[5,10] RV enlargement is evident on CTA and echocardiogram. Symptoms may include severe dyspnea, lightheadedness, syncope, and cyanosis. Physical examination may reveal tachypnea as well as tachycardia and signs of acute RV dysfunction, including distended neck veins, RV heave, an accentuated P2, and a tricuspid regurgitation murmur.

Altered mentation, acute kidney injury, and hepatic dysfunction are often seen.[5,10] Frequently, hemodynamic support with fluids and pressors is necessary. Ultimately, this clinical syndrome has a poor prognosis as it is associated with an increased risk of adverse outcomes, including cardiac arrest and death.[10]

Submassive PE represents another clinical syndrome in the spectrum of acute PE. The criteria that define it include normotension with acute PE and evidence of RV dysfunction. The presence of RV dysfunction can be identified by signs on physical examination, electrocardiographic evidence of RV strain, cardiac biomarker elevation (troponin and brain-type natriuretic peptide), echocardiographic evidence of RV dilatation and hypokinesis, and detection of RV enlargement on chest CT.[11] If no prior cardiopulmonary disease exists, these patients may in fact appear clinically well.[5] Nonetheless, patients with submassive PE may still go on to develop systemic arterial hypotension and deteriorate to cardiogenic shock over the course of several hours to days.[11] However, most patients survive, although escalation of care with hemodynamic support (fluids and pressors) and/or mechanical ventilation may ultimately become necessary.[5,11]

PATHOPHYSIOLOGY
Hemodynamics

The RV response to massive and submassive acute PE is dependent on a few factors: the extent of the emboli, the patient's underlying cardiopulmonary status, and the release of vasoactive and bronchoactive agents such as serotonin from platelets.[12–14] The extent of pulmonary arterial obstruction to blood flow plays a critical role in compromising physiology and predicting the degree of RV dysfunction.[12,15,16] In addition to physical obstruction, there is an increase in pulmonary vascular resistance in acute PE as a result of the release of pulmonary artery vasoconstrictors and hypoxemia (hypoxic vasoconstriction),[13] which in turn leads to an increase in RV afterload that can result in RV strain and hemodynamic compromise.[13,15] More specifically, the abrupt increase in RV afterload increases RV wall tension and leads to a dilated and hypokinetic right ventricle, thereby impairing RV systolic function.[13,15] Annular dilation of the tricuspid valve with associated tricuspid regurgitation also results from increased RV afterload.[13,15] In addition, the increased wall stress from RV pressure overload combined with decreases in cardiac output and perfusion pressures (due to compression of the right coronary artery and resultant diminished subendocardial perfusion) alters the equilibrium between myocardial oxygen supply and demand, thus potentially leading to ischemia and even infarction.[15,17] RV pressure overload also leads to interventricular septal flattening and with compromise of the left ventricle in diastole (interventricular dependence), impairing of left ventricular filling, resulting in diastolic dysfunction.[13,15,18] Overall, these alterations in RV mechanics result in decreased right-sided output (RV failure), reduced left ventricular preload, and subsequently diminished systemic cardiac output leading to hypotension or hemodynamic collapse.[15,19] As this pathologic process evolves, patients may maintain hemodynamic stability with a normal systemic blood pressure initially; but, this is often suddenly followed by rapid progression to systemic arterial hypotension and cardiac arrest.[17]

Impaired Gas Exchange

Gas exchange abnormalities are also seen as a result of acute PE. Most commonly, arterial hypoxemia (decreased Pa_{O_2}) with an increase in the alveolar-arterial oxygen difference is evident.[13] Other mechanisms that lead to impaired gas exchange include ventilation-perfusion mismatch (as blood flow from obstructed pulmonary arteries is redirected to other gas exchange units), increased total dead space (anatomic and physiologic dead space), and right-to-left shunting.[13] Hypocapnia and respiratory alkalosis may result from hyperventilation.[13] However, massive acute PE can also lead to hypercapnia as a result of significant increases in total dead space along with impaired minute ventilation.[13]

EXPERIMENTAL PE AND THE RV RESPONSE

Murine experimental models have been used extensively to study the pathophysiology of RV dysfunction in acute PE. Sullivan and colleagues[20] published a study in 2001 looking at biventricular dysfunction in the ex vivo perfused hearts of rats induced with acute massive PE via thrombus infusion. Their data (through examination of Starling curves) support the idea that the intrinsic mechanical function of both ventricles can become depressed in response to an acute massive PE (reduced RV systolic contractile function [$P = .031$] and reduced left ventricular systolic contractile function [$P = .008$]).[20] Furthermore, they surmise that their data support the hypothesis that biventricular depression, and not just RV collapse, may play important roles in the acute hemodynamic compromise that is seen in severe PE.[20]

Other studies have used murine experimental models of acute PE to focus on the gene expression changes within the heart following PE. Using DNA microarray analysis, Zagorski and colleagues[21] showed an increased expression of cytokine-induced neutrophil chemoattractant-1 (CINC-1) and CINC-2 between 6 and 18 hours after PE. Neutrophils, which in acute PE normally accumulate in the right ventricle by 18 hours and are associated with RV dysfunction, were significantly reduced after treatment of rats with antibodies to CINC-1.[21] Moreover, there was an improvement in RV failure, and the plasma concentration level of plasma troponin was drastically reduced.[21] Therefore, this study suggests that after PE, inhibition of neutrophilic chemoattractants such as CINC-1 can reduce inflammation in the right heart and preserve RV function.

The effect of prostaglandin synthesis inhibition on pulmonary gas exchange and cardiac function has also been studied during simulated PE in the rat. Jones and colleagues[22] performed a randomized blinded study of rats with induced fixed pulmonary vascular occlusion using polystyrene microspheres and showed increased production of thromboxane B_2 in the lung and systemically. More importantly, it was demonstrated that both thromboxane synthase inhibition (furegrelate sodium) and cyclooxygenase-1/2 inhibition (ketorolac tromethamine) significantly decreased the alveolar dead space fraction and improved right heart function in this rat model.[22]

Other such experimental PE studies are found in the literature and continue to provide insight on the pathophysiology of acute massive and submassive PE.

DIAGNOSTIC APPROACHES
Clinical Manifestations

It is critically important to prevent diagnostic and management delays when it comes to acute PE, particularly when the emboli are submassive or massive. Thus, having a clinical suspicion of PE is crucial in guiding diagnostic testing. Dyspnea, tachypnea, and tachycardia are the most common symptoms and signs of PE. In massive PE, severe dyspnea, syncope, and cyanosis can accompany hypotension, portending a poor prognosis.[5,13] Interestingly, significant pleuritic chest pain often signifies the presence of a smaller and more distally located embolism and not the more life-threatening moderate to large clots that are centrally located.[5] Other clinical signs of acute RV failure include tachycardia, distended neck veins, loud P_2, right-sided S_3 gallop, tricuspid regurgitation, and an RV heave.[5,12,13] Although symptoms and signs of both deep vein thrombosis (DVT) and PE may be highly suggestive, they are neither sensitive nor specific.[12] Thus, when VTE is suspected, further diagnostic testing must be considered.

Electrocardiogram

Electrocardiographic manifestations of right heart strain ($S_1Q_3T_3$ pattern, right bundle-branch block, P-wave pulmonale, or right axis deviation) are more common with massive embolism than with smaller emboli. However, all of these findings are nonspecific.[12,23] Patients with massive PE may have sinus tachycardia, slight ST- and T-wave abnormalities (anterior precordium), or even an entirely normal electrocardiogram.[5] Importantly, the potential for acute myocardial infarction can be evaluated.

Laboratory Testing

In an appropriately selected patient, exclusion of PE may be possible with D-dimer testing.[13] D-dimer is a break down product of fibrinolysis, and its elevation indicates the possibility of VTE.[12,13] However, although an elevated plasma D-dimer is sensitive for the presence of PE, it is nonspecific because it can also be elevated in almost any other systemic illness.[12] Thus, D-dimer testing is best used when considered together with pretest clinical probability.[12] When the enzyme-linked immunosorbent assay-based D-dimer test result is negative in patients with a low or moderate pretest probability, the likelihood of DVT and PE is exceedingly low and precludes the need for specific imaging studies.[12,24,25] This test, however, is not as useful in the acutely ill hospitalized patient, and it has no role in the diagnostic approach taken with individuals who have a high pretest probability of thromboembolic disease in which case radiographic imaging is indicated.[5,12]

Cardiac biomarkers are other clinically useful laboratory tests. They can assist with risk stratification once the diagnosis of acute PE has already been established.[12,15,26] Specifically, elevated levels of cardiac troponin, BNP, and pro-BNP may suggest the presence of RV failure in a patient with acute submassive or massive PE.[15,27–36] RV ischemia or infarction in the setting of increased RV wall tension and decreased perfusion pressures results in release of cardiac troponins into the circulation.[15,27] Increased RV shear stress in the acutely decompensated right ventricle is responsible for the synthesis and secretion of BNP from the myocardium.[15,27]

Imaging Studies

Many imaging modalities have been used in the evaluation of patients with suspected PE. The chest radiograph is often normal. Rare radiographic findings include focal oligemia (Westermark sign), a peripheral wedge-shaped opacity (Hampton hump), or an enlarged right descending pulmonary artery (Pallas sign).[5,13] Contrast-enhanced CT arteriography is currently the imaging test of choice for evaluating a suspected PE.[5,13] It has the greatest sensitivity and specificity for detecting emboli in the main, lobar, or segmental pulmonary arteries.[12] The newer multidetector CT scanners have markedly improved visualization of segmental and subsegmental vessels, thus increasing the detection rate.[12,13,37]

Ventilation-perfusion (VQ) lung scanning is generally reserved for patients with normal chest radiographs or contraindications to a contrasted chest CT study namely, renal insufficiency, anaphylaxis to intravenous contrast, or pregnancy.[13] The VQ scan is most likely to be diagnostic in the absence of underlying cardiopulmonary disease.[12,38] Magnetic resonance angiography (MRA) can also be used as a tool for detecting PE (particularly in the proximal pulmonary arteries).[13] However, it is less sensitive than CT for the detection of PE.[5] Major advantages of using an MRA include avoiding the risks of iodinated contrast and ionizing radiation.[5,13] In addition, it can assess RV size and function.[5]

Echocardiography is not used as a routine diagnostic tool for the detection of PE, given its lack of sensitivity.[5,13] However, it plays an important role in risk stratifying patients with known acute PE, thus offering the potential to guide therapy.[13] In moderate and large PE with resultant RV pressure overload, transthoracic echocardiography allows the assessment of RV dysfunction.[13] These findings include RV dilatation and hypokinesis, interventricular septal flattening and deviation toward the left ventricle, tricuspid regurgitation, and evidence of pulmonary hypertension.[13,39] McConnell sign, characterized by severe RV wall hypokinesis sparing the apex (regional RV dysfunction), is an echocardiographic finding that appears specific for PE.[13,40] Echo is also useful in detecting a patent foramen ovale as well as free-floating thrombus in the right side of the heart, which help identify patients at higher risk of death or recurrent thromboembolism.[5] Finally, echocardiography can help identify conditions that can mimic acute PE, such as myocardial infarction, aortic dissection, and pericardial disease.[5,13,15]

Fig. 1A demonstrates acute PE by CTA. Fig. 1B shows the relative size of the right and left ventricles in the same patient. Fig. 1C demonstrates extensive bilateral PE. Fig. 1D shows the severely enlarged right ventricle with septal bowing of the same patient, compromising the left ventricle.

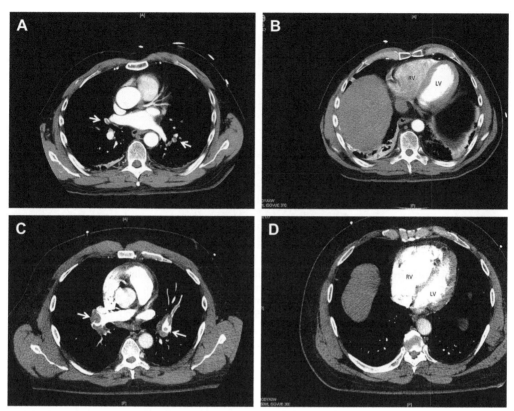

Fig. 1. (*A*) Bilateral PE predominantly affecting distal lobar vessels and segmental pulmonary arteries (*arrows*). (*B*) The same patient as in **Fig. 1**A. The right ventricle (RV) is upper limits of normal in size, with no septal bowing. The left ventricle (LV) is normal. This was confirmed on echocardiography. (*C*) Extensive bilateral PE (*arrows*). (*D*) The same patient as in **Fig. 1**C. Severely enlarged RV with septal bowing, compromising the LV.

Fig. 2 demonstrates echocardiographic findings in acute massive PE.

MANAGEMENT
Massive PE

Given its poor prognostic implications, it is imperative to act quickly whenever massive PE is suspected. Intravenous unfractionated heparin (weight-based protocol) should be bolused immediately, followed by continuous infusion of unfractionated heparin targeting an activated partial thromboplastin time (aPTT) of at least 80 seconds.[5,10,26] Although low-molecular-weight heparin can be used, the shorter half life of standard heparin may be advantageous if thrombolytic therapy, with its inherent bleeding risk is administered. Hemodynamic support with rapid volume resuscitation should be attempted. However, extreme caution should be observed so as not to administer excessive fluids (no more than 500–1000 mL normal saline), as this can worsen RV failure by exacerbating RV wall stress, intensifying RV ischemia, and causing further interventricular septal shift toward the left ventricle.[5,10,15,16,41–43] There

should be a low threshold for initiation of pressors (vasopressors and inotropes) to maintain adequate hemodynamic support.[10,15,16,41]

Thrombolytic therapy is recommended as a standard, first-line treatment in massive PE, unless there are major contraindications owing to bleeding risk (Grade 1B).[5,10,26,44–46] Tissue plasminogen activator (t-PA) has been approved by the FDA for treatment of massive PE, at a dose of 100 mg as a continuous infusion over 2 hours.[5,10,26,44–46] Heparin should be discontinued as soon as the decision is made to use alteplase.[5,10,26,44–46] At the conclusion of the infusion of the fibrinolytic agent, the aPTT should be checked, and if it is less than 80 seconds, intravenous heparin should be restarted as a continuous infusion without a bolus.[5,10,26,44–46] Reports have indicated that thrombolytic therapy for acute PE may offer the most benefit when given within the first few days of symptom onset, although enhanced clot lysis may still be observed when administered up to 2 weeks after an acute event.[46,47] If major contraindications exist and systemic thrombolysis is too risky, then consideration must be given to placement of an inferior vena cava filter, catheter embolectomy,

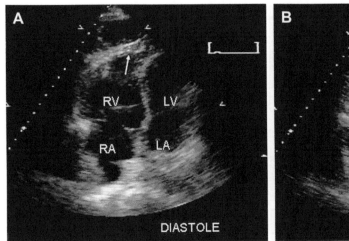
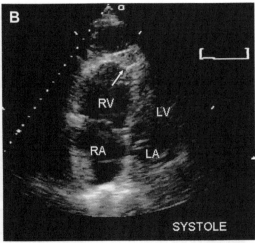

Fig. 2. Echocardiographic 4-chamber views of a patient with massive PE and RV dysfunction in end-diastole (*A*) and in end-systole (*B*). Arrows indicate normally contracting apical segments in a globally hypokinetic right ventricle (McConnell sign). LA, left atrium; LV, left ventricle; RA, right atrium, and RV, right ventricle. (*From* Casazza F, Bongarzoni A, Capozi A, et al. Regional right ventricular dysfunction in acute pulmonary embolism and right ventricular infarction. Eur J Echocardiogr 2005;6[1]:11–4; with permission.)

or surgical embolectomy.[5,10,26,45] Oxygen supplementation, intubation, and mechanical ventilation should be instituted as needed for respiratory failure.

Submassive PE

The treatment approach to submassive PE is less clear. Anticoagulation remains to be the cornerstone of therapy.[11,26,44–46] Addition of thrombolysis, inferior vena cava filter placement, and embolectomy remain controversial.[11,26,44–46] Bleeding complications are the major concern with thrombolysis in the setting of submassive PE, particularly if this fear outweighs any potential benefit.[11,26,44–46] The American College of Chest Physicians advises the following: "In selected high-risk patients without hypotension who are judged to have a low risk of bleeding, we suggest administration of thrombolytic therapy (Grade 2B)."[44] Thus, given the current lack of published data or adequate study trials, the decision to treat with anticoagulation alone or advancing therapy with lytics must be made on a case by case basis. There is a large, ongoing, multicenter, randomized controlled trial in Europe (Pulmonary Embolism International Thrombolysis Trial) that is studying thrombolytic therapy in high-risk normotensive PE patients, and it is planning to enroll approximately 1000 patients.[5,11] All-cause mortality and hemodynamic collapse within 7 days of treatment with a fibrinolytic agent (tenecteplase) plus heparin versus heparin alone will be their primary clinical endpoint.[5,11] It is hoped that this ambitious study will help clarify a more standardized treatment strategy.

Catheter-Based Therapies

The guidelines published by the European Society of Cardiology Task Force indicate that "catheter embolectomy or fragmentation of proximal pulmonary arterial clots may be considered as an alternative to surgical treatment in high-risk PE patients when thrombolysis is absolutely contraindicated or has failed."[48] Three general categories of catheter-based interventions are (1) aspiration embolectomy, (2) catheter-directed embolus fragmentation, and (3) rheolysis.[49,50] Aspiration embolectomy has used the Greenfield suction embolectomy catheter (Boston Scientific/Meditech; Watertown, MA) to secure and extract the clot using sustained suction at the catheter tip.[49,50] Catheter-directed embolus fragmentation can be performed with various catheter devices that break apart large proximal emboli by direct mechanical action.[49] Most results reported on these devices have also included local thrombolysis. Catheter-based rheolysis is achieved through the use of devices that use high-velocity injection creating a vortex or high-pressure saline jets, resulting in fragmentation of the thrombus.[49,50] The fragmented debris is then collected and evacuated.[49,50] Finally, the novel concept of the use of ultrasonic devices to gently accelerate the penetration of thrombolytic agents into thrombus has been studied and seems beneficial.[51]

Importantly, the guidelines make it clear that only experienced operators should perform catheter-based interventions.[50] The recent 2011 American Heart Association Scientific Statement[50] recommends the following: "Depending on local expertise, either catheter embolectomy and fragmentation or surgical embolectomy is reasonable for patients with massive PE and contraindications to fibrinolysis (Class IIa; Level of Evidence C)." The statement also states that "for patients with massive PE who cannot receive fibrinolysis or who remain unstable after fibrinolysis, it is reasonable to consider transfer to an institution experienced in either catheter embolectomy or surgical embolectomy if these procedures are not available locally and safe transfer can be achieved (Class IIa; Level of Evidence C).[50]

SUMMARY

It is critically important to quickly recognize and treat acute PE. Submassive and massive PE are associated with RV dysfunction and may culminate in RV failure, cardiac arrest, and death. The normally thin-walled right ventricle is a conduit that acutely cannot hold up to the abrupt increase in RV afterload following an extensive PE, and the resultant high RV pressure overload is crucial in appreciating the clinicopathologic progression of this disease. Ultimately, a rapid and coordinated diagnostic and management approach can maximize success and save lives.

CLINICAL CASE (CONTINUED)

Several hours after admission to the hospital ward, the patient became hypotensive (BP 82/46). This hypotension did not respond to a normal saline bolus (1000 mL). His clinical deterioration further progressed and oxygen requirements increased; he ultimately required a 100% non-rebreather mask to maintain his oxygen saturation above 90%. Pressors were initiated, and the medical team agreed to treat with thrombolytic therapy. Recombinant t-PA was infused for 2 hours, and during this time his blood pressure improved and was ultimately weaned off of pressors. Fortunately, intubation was avoided and he had no bleeding complications. Heparin was resumed and then changed to enoxaparin. After 10 days in the hospital, the patient was discharged with an enoxaparin bridge to warfarin therapy. At his 1-month follow-up, his symptoms and oxygenation had returned to normal. A repeat echocardiogram performed immediately before this follow-up visit demonstrated normal RV size and function.

REFERENCES

1. Silverstein MD, Heit JA, Mohr DN, et al. Trends in the incidence of deep vein thrombosis and pulmonary embolism: a 25-year population-based study. Arch Intern Med 1998;158:585–93.
2. Heit JA, Cohen AT, Anderson FA, et al. Estimated annual number of incident and recurrent, non-fatal and fatal venous thromboembolism (VTE) events in the US [abstract]. Blood 2005;106:267a.
3. Sandler DA, Martin JF. Autopsy proven pulmonary embolism in hospital patients: are we detecting enough deep vein thrombosis? J R Soc Med 1989;82:203–5.
4. Bergqvist D, Lindblad B. A 30-year survey of pulmonary embolism verified at autopsy: an analysis of 1274 surgical patients. Br J Surg 1985;72:105–8.
5. Goldhaber SZ. Pulmonary embolism. In: Bonow RO, Mann DL, Zipes DP, et al, editors. Braunwald's heart disease: a textbook of cardiovascular medicine. 9th edition. Philadelphia: Saunders; 2011. p. 1679–95.
6. Goldhaber SZ, Visani L, De Rosa M. Acute pulmonary embolism: clinical outcomes in the International Cooperative Pulmonary Embolism Registry (ICOPER). Lancet 1999;353:1386–9.
7. Heit JA. The epidemiology of venous thromboembolism in the community: implications for prevention and management. J Thromb Thrombolysis 2006;21:23–9.
8. Piazza G, Seddighzadeh A, Goldhaber SZ. Double trouble for 2,609 hospitalized medical patients who developed deep vein thrombosis: prophylaxis omitted more often and pulmonary embolism more frequent. Chest 2007;132(2):554–61.
9. Schreijer AJ, Cannegieter SC, Meijers JC, et al. Activation of coagulation system during air travel: a crossover study. Lancet 2006;367:832–8.
10. Kucher N, Goldhaber SZ. Management of massive pulmonary embolism. Circulation 2005;112:e28–32.
11. Piazza G, Goldhaber SZ. Management of submassive pulmonary embolism. Circulation 2010;122:1124–9.
12. Tapson VF. Acute pulmonary embolism. N Engl J Med 2008;358:1037–52.
13. Piazza G, Goldhaber SZ. Acute pulmonary embolism, part I: epidemiology and diagnosis. Circulation 2006;114:e28–32.
14. Elliott CG. Pulmonary physiology during pulmonary embolism. Chest 1992;101(Suppl 4):163S–71S.
15. Piazza G, Goldhaber SZ. The acutely decompensated right ventricle. Chest 2005;128:1836–52.
16. Lualdi JC, Goldhaber SZ. Right ventricular dysfunction after acute pulmonary embolism: pathophysiologic factors, detection, and therapeutic implications. Am Heart J 1995;130:1276–82.
17. Goldhaber SZ, Elliott G. Acute pulmonary embolism: part I, epidemiology, pathophysiology, and diagnosis. Circulation 2003;108:2726–9.
18. Jardin F, Dubourg O, Gueret P, et al. Quantitative two-dimensional echocardiography in massive pulmonary embolism: emphasis on ventricular interdependence and leftward septal displacement. J Am Coll Cardiol 1987;10:1201–6.

19. Pfisterer M. Right ventricular involvement in myocardial infarction and cardiogenic shock. Lancet 2003; 362:392–4.

20. Sullivan DM, Watts JA, Kline JA. Biventricular cardiac dysfunction after acute massive pulmonary embolism in the rat. J Appl Physiol 2001;90:1648–56.

21. Zagorski J, Gellar MA, Obraztsova M, et al. Inhibition of CINC-1 decreases right ventricular damage caused by experimental pulmonary embolism in rats. J Immunol 2007;179:7820–6.

22. Jones AE, Watts JA, Debelak JP, et al. Inhibition of prostaglandin synthesis during polystyrene microsphere-induced pulmonary embolism in the rat. Am J Physiol Lung Cell Mol Physiol 2003;284:L1072–81.

23. Stein PD, Terrin ML, Hales CA, et al. Clinical, laboratory, roentgenographic, and electrocardiographic findings in patients with acute pulmonary embolism and no pre-existing cardiac or pulmonary disease. Chest 1991;100:598–603.

24. Di Nisio M, Squizzato A, Rutjes AW, et al. Diagnostic accuracy of D-dimer test for exclusion of venous thromboembolism: a systematic review. J Thromb Haemost 2007;5:296–304.

25. Kearon C, Ginsberg JS, Douketis J, et al. An evaluation of D-dimer in the diagnosis of pulmonary embolism: a randomized trial. Ann Intern Med 2006; 144:812–21.

26. Piazza G, Goldhaber SZ. Acute pulmonary embolism, part II: treatment and prophylaxis. Circulation 2006;114:e42–7.

27. Kucher N, Goldhaber SZ. Cardiac biomarkers for risk stratification of patients with acute pulmonary embolism. Circulation 2003;108:2191–4.

28. Konstantinides S, Geibel A, Olschewski M, et al. Importance of cardiac troponins I and T in risk stratification of patients with acute pulmonary embolism. Circulation 2002;106:1263–8.

29. Giannitsis E, Muller-Bardorff M, Kurowski V, et al. Independent prognostic value of cardiac troponin T in patients with confirmed pulmonary embolism. Circulation 2000;102:211–7.

30. Janata K, Holzer M, Laggner AN, et al. Cardiac troponin T in the severity assessment of patients with pulmonary embolism: cohort study. BMJ 2003; 326:312–3.

31. Pruszczyk P, Kostrubiec M, Bochowicz A, et al. N-terminal pro-brain natriuretic peptide in patients with acute pulmonary embolism. Eur Respir J 2003;22:649–53.

32. Pruszczyk P, Bochowicz A, Torbicki A, et al. Cardiac troponin T monitoring identifies high-risk group of normotensive patients with acute pulmonary embolism. Chest 2003;123:1947–52.

33. Meyer T, Binder L, Hruska N, et al. Cardiac troponin I elevation in acute pulmonary embolism is associated with right ventricular dysfunction. J Am Coll Cardiol 2000;36:1632–6.

34. Kucher N, Printzen G, Goldhaber SZ. Prognostic role of brain natriuretic peptide in acute pulmonary embolism. Circulation 2003;107:2545–7.

35. Kucher N, Printzen G, Doernhoefer T, et al. Low probrain natriuretic peptide levels predict benign clinical outcome in acute pulmonary embolism. Circulation 2003;107:1576–8.

36. ten Wolde M, Tulevski II, Mulder JW, et al. Brain natriuretic peptide as a predictor of adverse outcome in patients with pulmonary embolism. Circulation 2003; 107:2082–4.

37. Schoepf UJ, Holzknecht N, Helmberger TK, et al. Subsegmental pulmonary emboli: improved detection with thin-collimation multidetector row spiral CT. Radiology 2002;222:483–90.

38. The PIOPED Investigators. Value of the ventilation/perfusion scan in acute pulmonary embolism: results of the Prospective Investigation of Pulmonary Embolism Diagnosis (PIOPED). JAMA 1990;263: 2753–9.

39. Goldhaber SZ. Echocardiography in the management of pulmonary embolism. Ann Intern Med 2002;136:691–700.

40. McConnell MV, Solomon SD, Rayan ME, et al. Regional right ventricular dysfunction detected by echocardiography in acute pulmonary embolism. Am J Cardiol 1996;78:469–73.

41. Layish DT, Tapson VF. Pharmacologic hemodynamic support in massive pulmonary embolism. Chest 1997;111:218–24.

42. Mercat A, Diehl JL, Meyer G, et al. Hemodynamic effects of fluid loading in acute massive pulmonary embolism. Crit Care Med 1999;27:540–4.

43. Wood KE. Major pulmonary embolism: review of a pathophysiologic approach to the golden hour of hemodynamically significant pulmonary embolism. Chest 2002;121:877–905.

44. Kearon C, Kahn SR, Agnelli G, et al. Antithrombotic therapy for venous thromboembolic disease: American College of Chest Physicians Evidence-Based Clinical Practice Guidelines (8th Edition). Chest 2008;133(Suppl 6):454S–545S.

45. Piazza G, Goldhaber SZ. Fibrinolysis for acute pulmonary embolism. Vasc Med 2010;15(5):419–28.

46. Todd JL, Tapson VF. Thrombolytic therapy for acute pulmonary embolism: a critical appraisal. Chest 2009;135(5):1321–9.

47. Daniels LB, Parker JA, Patel SR, et al. Relation of duration of symptoms with response to thrombolytic therapy in pulmonary embolism. Am J Cardiol 1997; 80:184–8.

48. Torbicki A, Perrier A, Konstantinides S, et al. Guidelines on the diagnosis and management of acute pulmonary embolism. The Task Force for the Diagnosis and Management of Acute Pulmonary Embolism of the European Society of Cardiology (ESC). Eur Heart J 2008;29:2276–315.

49. Tapson VF. Interventional therapies for venous thromboembolism: vena caval interruption, surgical embolectomy, and catheter-directed interventions. Clin Chest Med 2010;31:771–81.
50. Jaff MR, McMurtry MS, Archer SL, et al. Management of massive and submassive pulmonary embolism, iliofemoral deep vein thrombosis, and chronic thromboembolic pulmonary hypertension: a scientific statement from the American Heart Association. Circulation 2011;123:1788–830.
51. Stambo GW, Montague B. Bilateral EKOS EndoWave™ catheter thrombolysis of acute bilateral pulmonary embolism in a hemodynamically unstable patient. South Med J 2010;3:455–7.

Right Ventricular Dysfunction in Chronic Lung Disease

Todd M. Kolb, MD, PhD[a], Paul M. Hassoun, MD[a,b,*]

KEYWORDS

- Right ventricle • Pulmonary hypertension • Cor pulmonale
- Chronic lung disease

Key Points

- The prevalence of pulmonary hypertension and right ventricular remodeling is variable in chronic lung disease but increases with disease progression.
- Chronic hypoxemia and disruption of pulmonary vascular beds contribute to increase pulmonary vascular resistance and promote right ventricular remodeling.
- Right ventricular contractility is generally preserved in chronic lung disease.
- Right ventricular dysfunction can be difficult to distinguish noninvasively from underlying progression of pulmonary disease.
- Correction of hypoxia with long term oxygen therapy and pulmonary disease-specific therapies are the mainstay of treatment.
- Pulmonary hypertension–specific therapies have not shown benefit in right ventricular dysfunction associated with chronic lung disease and may worsen hypoxia.
- Development of pulmonary hypertension and right ventricular dysfunction worsens survival in chronic lung disease.
- Right ventricular failure is rare except during acute exacerbations of chronic lung disease or when multiple comorbidities are present.

NATURE OF THE PROBLEM

Nearly 200 years ago, Laennec described the relationship between chronic pulmonary disease and right ventricular (RV) dysfunction: "All diseases which give rise to severe and long-continued dyspnœa produced, almost necessarily, hypertrophia or dilatation of the heart, through the constant efforts the organ is called on to perform, to propel the blood into the lungs against the resistance opposed to it by the cause of the dyspnœa".[1] Our understanding of cardio-pulmonary pathophysiology has increased exponentially since that publication, although Laennec's basic observation concisely described the essence of RV dysfunction in chronic lung disease. Structural changes of the lung parenchyma and functional abnormalities in gas exchange lead to pulmonary hypertension

---

Supported by National Heart, Lung and Blood Institute grants P50 HL084946 (P.H.) and F32 HL 110516 (T.K.). The authors have nothing to disclose.

[a] Division of Pulmonary and Critical Care Medicine, Johns Hopkins University, 1830 East Monument Street, 5th Floor, Baltimore, MD 21205, USA; [b] Pulmonary Hypertension Program, Johns Hopkins University, 1830 East Monument Street, 5th Floor, Baltimore, MD 21205, USA
* Corresponding author. Division of Pulmonary and Critical Care Medicine, Johns Hopkins University, 1830 East Monument Street, 5th Floor, Baltimore, MD 21205.
E-mail address: phassou1@jhmi.edu

Cardiol Clin 30 (2012) 243–256
doi:10.1016/j.ccl.2012.03.005
0733-8651/12/$ – see front matter © 2012 Elsevier Inc. All rights reserved

(PH), with subsequent RV remodeling and hypertrophy. The term cor pulmonale was used to describe this relationship, although the importance of PH was not emphasized.[2] More recently, several disorders associated with chronic lung disease or hypoxia have been grouped together in the classification of PH.[3] In general, these disorders are characterized by mild PH, and RV dysfunction is characterized by hypertrophy with preserved cardiac function. However, RV failure can occur during disease exacerbations or when multiple comorbidities are present, and the development of PH increases mortality in many chronic pulmonary conditions.

The current review focuses on World Health Organization Group 3 disorders (**Box 1**), with primary attention to chronic obstructive pulmonary disease (COPD), interstitial lung disease (ILD), and sleep disordered breathing (SDB), because these account for the bulk of cases. COPD is estimated to account for approximately 80% of Group 3 disease.[4,5] Other diseases, including sarcoidosis, pulmonary Langerhans cell histiocytosis, and scleroderma-associated lung disease, can produce both parenchymal lung disease and pulmonary hypertension, but given their complex effects on the pulmonary vasculature they are not grouped with other chronic lung diseases in the most recent PH classification.[3]

Prevalence of PH in Chronic Lung Disease

The prevalence of PH in chronic lung disease has been difficult to quantify because of the limited population-based hemodynamic data available and variability in the definition used to identify PH in these patients. Chronic lung disease seems to be a common comorbidity in patients with PH

Box 1
Chronic lung diseases associated with pulmonary hypertension and right ventricular dysfunction

- Chronic obstructive pulmonary disease
- Interstitial lung disease
- Mixed obstructive and restrictive lung disease
- Sleep-disordered breathing
- Alveolar hypoventilation disorders
- Chronic exposure to high altitude
- Developmental abnormalities

Data from Simonneau G, Robbins IM, Beghetti M, et al. Updated clinical classification of pulmonary hypertension. J Am Coll Cardiol 2009;54:S45.

---

and was present in 25.9% of all patients who died from pulmonary hypertension in the United States between 2000 and 2002.[6] Prevalence estimates for PH in COPD range from 30% to 70%,[7] with PH being more common in patients with advanced disease. In one trial of patients with severe emphysema evaluated for lung volume reduction surgery, 61.4% of patients had a mean pulmonary artery (PA) pressure greater than 20 mm Hg.[8] Because this value represents the upper limit of normal resting mean PA pressure[9] most investigators have used this value to define PH in chronic lung disease, despite the higher mean PA pressure required to define pulmonary arterial hypertension. The prevalence of PH and RV dysfunction in other obstructive lung diseases, including asthma, cystic fibrosis, bronchiolitis obliterans, and bronchiectasis is less clear. Prevalence estimates for ILD-associated PH are even more variable (8%–84%), probably because of the heterogeneous nature of these disorders.[10]

Pulmonary hypertension prevalence increases with the severity of ILD: from 8.1% in patients with idiopathic pulmonary fibrosis (IPF) at initial evaluation[11] to 30% to 40% in patients with IPF at the time of transplant evaluation or referral to tertiary care.[12,13] Obstructive sleep apnea (OSA) has been associated with PH prevalence estimates of 20% to 40%,[14] although other comorbidities frequently confound the diagnosis. One study estimated that PH prevalence in isolated OSA with all other restrictive and obstructive lung disease excluded was 9%, whereas the prevalence of PH in patients with obesity hypoventilation syndrome (OHS) was nearly 58%.[15]

PATHOPHYSIOLOGY
Effects of Chronic Pulmonary Disease on Right Heart Structure and Function

Hypertrophy of the RV with preserved systolic function is the predominant effect of chronic pulmonary disease. Chronic pulmonary disease results in fairly slow increases in PA pressure (about 3 mm Hg/year[16]), allowing time for adequate compensation. The normally thin-walled, compliant RV is hypertrophied to mitigate intraluminal pressure increases and ultimately minimizes wall stress. Increased RV thickness is accompanied by hypertrophy of individual myocytes, remodeling of the myocardial extracellular matrix, alterations in glucose metabolism, and in some models, compensatory increases in capillary density.[17–19]

Concentric RV hypertrophy can precede resting hypoxia in patients with stable COPD[20] and was demonstrated at autopsy in 76% of patients with advanced COPD.[21] RV hypertrophy was estimated to be present in 50% of patients with restrictive lung disease.[22] One study showed that 71% of patients with OSA had RV hypertrophy at echocardiography.[23] However, it remains unclear whether RV hypertrophy results from isolated OSA or other co-morbidities. Whereas RV wall thickness increased in subjects with SDB in the Framingham cohort,[24] a later study of OSA patients without pulmonary disease or evidence of LV dysfunction, showed no increase in RV wall thickness.[25]

Despite these changes in RV structure, myocardial systolic function is generally preserved in PH associated with chronic lung disease. Although earlier studies demonstrated that slight reductions in RV ejection fraction occurred commonly in chronic lung disease,[26] the dependence of ejection fraction on ventricular preload, afterload, and myocardial contractility made this observation difficult to interpret. Intrinsic myocardial contractility seems to be preserved in patients with COPD as demonstrated by the normal RV end-systolic pressure-volume relationship measured at rest and with exercise.[27,28] RV diastolic function may be impaired in patients with chronic lung disease and PH, as demonstrated by the direct associations between PH and reduced early to late ventricular filling velocity ratio (E/A ratio) and prolonged myocardial relaxation time in patients with COPD.[29] Impaired RV diastolic function can also be demonstrated in healthy individuals exposed to acute hypoxia.[30]

Effects of Chronic Pulmonary Disease on RV Afterload

Increased pulmonary vascular resistance (PVR) is the sine qua non of RV dysfunction in chronic pulmonary disease. Chronic hypoxemia and the disruption of pulmonary vascular beds through parenchymal loss and fibrosis are the key mechanisms through which chronic lung disease increases PVR.

Alveolar hypoxia induces rapid vasoconstriction of small precapillary pulmonary arteries to preserve the ventilation to perfusion (V/Q) ratio and minimize effects on arterial oxygen saturation. The mechanisms of hypoxic pulmonary vasoconstriction are reviewed elsewhere[31] and involve alterations in potassium and calcium flux in smooth muscle cells, resulting in contraction and increased vascular tone. Pulmonary vasoconstriction can be further exacerbated by hypercapnia and acidemia in COPD[32] or by increased sympathetic activity in OSA.[14] However, supplemental oxygen administration does not fully reverse the increased PA pressure observed in patients with COPD[33] and

correlations between PA pressure and systemic oxygenation have not been robust.[34] This probably reflects individual differences in the capacity for hypoxic pulmonary vasoconstriction and/or differences in pulmonary vascular remodeling in response to chronic hypoxia. Chronic hypoxia results in remodeling of the pulmonary vasculature, characterized by neo-muscularization of arterioles, medial hypertrophy of small muscular arteries, and intimal thickening and fibroelastosis.[35]

Systemic hypoxemia arises in chronic lung disease through diverse mechanisms. COPD is a chronic inflammatory disorder of small airways that leads to airflow limitation, impaired gas exchange, and parenchymal loss in the case of emphysema. Hypoxemia results from impaired V/Q matching and is compounded by the loss of alveolar surface area for diffusion in emphysema. Interstitial lung diseases represent a more heterogeneous group of disorders, characterized by inflammatory or fibrotic destruction of lung parenchyma, generally at the level of the alveolar interstitium. These changes may be associated with autoimmune disease, exposure to cigarette smoke and other respiratory irritants, granulomatous diseases, or may be idiopathic. Interstitial changes result in impaired diffusing capacity, which may be exacerbated by poor V/Q matching in some patients. In OSA, hypoxia results from hypoventilation during obstructive episodes and is by definition intermittent. However, in patients with OHS or an overlap syndrome of COPD and OSA, diurnal hypoxemia may be present. At altitude, pulmonary vascular remodeling induced by chronic alveolar hypoxia can be exacerbated by hypoventilation, resulting in chronic mountain sickness that is frequently associated with PH and right heart dysfunction.[36]

Another common factor in the increased PVR associated with chronic lung disease is the disruption of pulmonary capillary beds. In COPD, the loss of alveolated lung tissue that occurs in emphysema, may result in loss of pulmonary capillary beds. This finding is supported by the negative correlation observed between diffusing capacity for carbon monoxide (D_LCO) and mean PA pressure in patients with severe COPD.[37] Mechanical compression of extra-alveolar vessels by lung hyperinflation had been assumed to contribute to PVR but later evidence did not support this hypothesis.[38] In ILD, interstitial fibrosis and inflammatory infiltrates may promote the loss of pulmonary vascular beds and compression of small vessels. Vessel ablation is common within fibroblastic foci and areas of 'honeycombing'."[39] Pulmonary vessel capacitance may also be reduced by nearby fibrosis[39] or by compensatory proliferation of abnormal capillaries lacking normal elastin layers.[40] Thromboembolic lesions can further impede pulmonary vascular flow and they frequently complicate chronic lung diseases, such as COPD,[41,42] sarcoidosis,[43] and IPF.[44]

Effects of Chronic Pulmonary Disease on Cardiac Mechanics

Chronic pulmonary disease may alter right and left ventricular function by changing intrathoracic pressure. Lung hyperinflation may increase right atrial pressure, leading to reduced venous return and subsequent reductions in RV preload.[45] In patients with COPD, hyperinflation has been directly correlated with reduced atrial chamber size, global RV dysfunction, and reduced LV filling.[46] In addition, highly negative pleural pressures may be necessary to facilitate ventilation in COPD or during episodes of airway obstruction in OSA. These highly negative pleural pressures reduce intrathoracic pressure and increase LV wall stress during ejection,[47] potentially resulting in left atrial hypertension and increased RV afterload.

CLINICAL EVALUATION
Physical Examination

It can be difficult to distinguish chronic lung disease from associated PH and RV dysfunction. Increased exertional dyspnea may arise from new RV dysfunction or progression of the underlying parenchymal lung disease. Symptoms associated with advanced RV dysfunction (leg edema, ascites) may not be present, or may develop independently of RV dysfunction. In COPD, peripheral edema can develop as a consequence of chronic hypercapnia and renal vasoconstriction with activation of the renin-angiotensin-aldosterone system.[48] Peripheral edema is not a common occurrence in ILD patients with equivalent levels of hypoxemia, and is rare in COPD patients without hypercapnea.[48]

Physical signs may also be of limited value in the evaluation of chronic lung disease-associated PH and RV dysfunction. Classical signs of RV dysfunction, including a precordial heave, accentuated pulmonic component of S2, murmur of tricuspid regurgitation, or a right-sided gallop, may not be present in mild disease. Auscultatory findings may be limited by chest over-inflation (in COPD) and the abnormal pulmonary examination of most patients with parenchymal lung disease.

Non-Invasive Evaluation

Most noninvasive diagnostic modalities lack the sensitivity to identify new RV dysfunction in parenchymal lung disease. Electrocardiogram findings associated with RV dysfunction include a rightward P-wave axis, $S_1S_2S_3$ pattern, S_1Q_3 pattern, RV hypertrophy, and right bundle branch block.[10] ECG alone, however, is insensitive for the diagnosis of RV dysfunction. In one study of COPD patients with PH, abnormal ECG findings had a sensitivity of only 51%.[49]

Plain chest radiography findings associated with PH and RV remodeling may include enlarged central pulmonary arteries and the loss of the retrosternal air space. In patients with COPD, these radiographic abnormalities had a sensitivity of 46% and specificity of 63% in detecting PH.[49] However, on chest CT imaging, the enlargement of the main pulmonary artery to a diameter of 29 mm or greater was associated with high sensitivity (84%), specificity (75%), and positive predictive value (95%) in a heterogeneous group of patients with chronic lung disease.[50] However, CT findings may be less reliable in patients with IPF.[51]

Pulmonary function testing is necessary for the initial diagnosis of most chronic lung diseases that cause RV dysfunction and it provides objective evidence of disease progression or stability. Isolated reductions in $D_L CO$ have been associated with PH in IPF, sarcoidosis, and systemic sclerosis (SSc),[52–54] as shown in **Fig. 1**. However, a reduced $D_L CO$ is not predictive of elevated PA pressure in patients with COPD.[55] In patients with SSc, the distinction between pulmonary arterial hypertension and ILD-associated PH may be important in determining prognosis and response to therapeutics[56]; and the ratio of forced vital capacity/$D_L CO$ can predict pulmonary arterial hypertension in SSc patients with mild fibrotic lung disease.[57]

Assessment of exercise capacity may support a diagnosis of RV dysfunction in chronic lung disease. There is a modest negative correlation between the 6-minute walk distance (6MWD) and the estimated systolic PA pressure in patients with COPD.[55] Significant reductions in 6MWD have been reported in IPF patients with moderate to severe PH.[58] Cardiopulmonary exercise testing (CPET) may be more useful in the detection of increased PA pressure in patients with chronic lung disease.[59] Chronic lung disease-associated increases in PVR impair the normal exercise-induced pulmonary vasodilatory response, resulting in elevated PA pressure, increased V/Q mismatch and dead space ventilation, and reduced ventilatory efficiency (V_E/VCO_2). Progressive increases in V_E/VCO_2 and reductions in end-tidal CO_2 measurements with exercise, have been associated with secondary PH in COPD and ILD.[60–62]

Elevated plasma levels of brain natriuretic peptide (BNP) or N-terminal pro-brain natriuretic

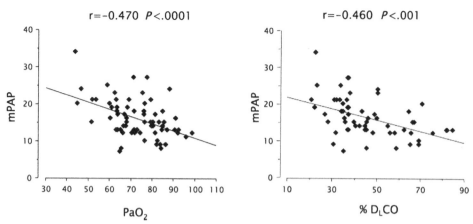

Fig. 1. Correlation of mean pulmonary arterial pressure (mPAP) with PaO_2 (left and percentage of predicted D_LCO [% D_LCO] right) in patients with idiopathic pulmonary fibrosis. (*From* Hamada K, Nagai S, Tanaka S, et al. Significance of pulmonary arterial pressure and diffusion capacity of the lung as prognosticator in patients with idiopathic pulmonary fibrosis. Chest 2007;131(3):650–6; with permission.)

peptide (NT-proBNP) are promising serologic markers that may suggest RV dysfunction in chronic lung disease. Natriuretic peptides are released from cardiac myocytes in response to increased wall stress; their serum levels must be interpreted with caution because they vary in populations based on age, gender, body mass index, and the presence of renal dysfunction.[10] However, elevated BNP levels were shown to predict PH in patients with chronic lung disease with a reasonably high sensitivity (85%) and specificity (88%).[63] In patients with COPD, BNP levels correlated with estimated PA pressure measurements even when patients were asymptomatic.[64]

Cardiac magnetic resonance imaging (cMRI) has been used increasingly to investigate the relationship between COPD and RV structure and function. cMRI has been used to show that concentric RV hypertrophy precedes RV dilatation in stable COPD patients without resting hypoxia,[20] and that exercise-induced increases in stroke volume are preload-dependent and limited by increases in PA pressure in patients with COPD.[65] Similarly, the MESA-Lung study[66] used cMRI to demonstrate that LV end-diastolic volumes and stroke volume are inversely correlated to percent emphysema, as detected by CT scan. Whereas cMRI holds great promise in furthering the understanding of RV structure and function in chronic lung disease, expense and limited availability make the technique somewhat impractical for routine clinical use. However, research findings have shown that volumes measured by electrocardiographically-gated cardiac CT imaging were well correlated with those obtained from cMRI,[67] and provide an

additional tool for clinical use that may be more widely available.

Transthoracic echocardiography is perhaps the best initial noninvasive study to assess RV function in chronic lung disease. The technique is noninvasive and allows for serial measurements over time. Two-dimensional estimates of RV chamber size, wall thickness, PA systolic pressure, and left heart function may be useful in the evaluation of PH in patients with chronic lung disease. However, image analysis is often limited by hyperinflation or parenchymal lung abnormalities. One study noted that a well-defined tricuspid regurgitant jet was present in only 20% of patients with chronic lung disease.[68] The correlation between estimated systolic PA pressure and pulmonary pressures measured by RHC is poor in advanced lung disease[69] and estimated PA pressures are insensitive for detection of PH in this patient population. In a study of patients with advanced COPD referred for lung volume reduction surgery, echocardiographic RV systolic pressure estimates detected PH with a sensitivity of only 60% and specificity of 74%.[70] Tricuspid annular plane systolic excursion (TAPSE) seems to be an accurate measure of RV function in patients with PH, including those with PH secondary to chronic respiratory disease.[71] This technique is not dependent on endocardial border recognition, which can be difficult in chronic lung disease patients. Newer techniques, including three-dimensional echocardiography, tissue Doppler ultrasonography, and ultrasound strain imaging may increase the potential for noninvasive assessment of the RV function in patients with chronic lung disease, and have been reviewed.[72]

Invasive Hemodynamic Measurements

Right heart catheterization (RHC) remains the gold standard in the assessment of PH, regardless of etiology. However, the procedure is invasive, costly, and requires performance by a skilled practitioner for safety and accurate interpretation. Given the generally mild hemodynamic changes in PH associated with pulmonary disease and the lack of evidence that PH-specific therapies provide benefit in this particular group (see later), RHC is not routinely recommended in this patient population. However, patients with chronic lung disease with clinical or echocardiographic evidence of advanced RV dysfunction out of proportion to their lung disease, might benefit from RHC, because severe PH or RV failure is usually associated with additional comorbidities. Generally, the degree of PH is mild in chronic lung disease, with mean PA pressures ranging from 20 mm Hg to 35 mm Hg.[5] In one large retrospective review of COPD patients undergoing RHC for lung transplant evaluation, 60% of the patients with a mean PA pressure greater than 40 mm Hg also

had some other precipitant (chronic thromboembolic disease, OSA, left ventricular disease).[73] RHC may also be indicated when patients are considered for lung transplantation, because the Lung Allocation Score emphasizes the presence of PH, particularly in ILD, thereby expediting organ allocation.[74]

THERAPEUTIC OPTIONS

In general, therapies to ameliorate RV dysfunction in chronic lung disease (**Table 1**) are targeted at mitigating the increased PVR associated with these conditions. Long term oxygen therapy (LTOT) and therapeutics targeted at the underlying pulmonary disease constitute the basis for therapy. There is limited evidence that medications targeting the pulmonary vasculature directly have any benefit in chronic lung disease.

Long Term Oxygen Therapy

The survival benefit of LTOT in chronic obstructive lung disease has been recognized from the early

Table 1
Therapeutic options for right ventricular dysfunction in chronic pulmonary disease

Therapy	Likely to Benefit
Long-term oxygen therapy	All patients with resting, ambulatory, or nocturnal hypoxemia
Diuretics	All patients with peripheral edema
Disease-specific therapy	
Smoking cessation	All patients
Pulmonary rehabilitation	All patients with advanced obstructive or restrictive lung disease
Inhaled bronchodilators, anticholinergics, and corticosteroids	Chronic obstructive pulmonary disease, asthma, other obstructive lung diseases
Systemic corticosteroids and other immunosuppressants	Unknown, potential benefit in sarcoidosis, pulmonary Langerhans cell histiocytosis
Weight loss	All patients with obesity
Uvulopalatopharyngoplasty	Patients with mild to moderate OSA
Nasal CPAP	All patients with sleep-disordered breathing
Pulmonary hypertension-specific therapy	
Inhaled nitric oxide	Chronic obstructive pulmonary disease
Phosphodiesterase-5 inhibitors	Unknown
Endothelin receptor antagonists	Unknown
Prostacyclin analogs	Unknown; may be of some benefit with inhaled formulation in COPD
Statins	Unknown
Surgical options	
Lung volume reduction surgery	None
Lung transplantation	Selected patients with severe parenchymal lung disease complicated by PH

1980s.[16,75] LTOT minimizes RV afterload in COPD, because patients using supplemental oxygen for at least 15 hours daily did not develop the increased PA pressure and PVR observed in patients with COPD who did not receive LTOT.[16] Later, LTOT was shown to stabilize the mean PA pressure in patients with severe COPD during a 6-year course, despite progressive declines in PaO_2 and FEV_1.[76] LTOT minimizes acute hypoxic pulmonary vasoconstriction and prevents further pulmonary vascular remodeling. Because pulmonary hemodynamic parameters stabilize but do not improve with LTOT, it is unlikely that pulmonary vascular remodeling is reversed.

In ILD, treatment of hypoxia with LTOT is widely accepted although it is not evidence-based. No studies have identified survival benefit for LTOT in patients with ILD.[77] Supplemental oxygen therapy should be titrated carefully in ILD patients, because growing evidence supports a role for hyperoxia-mediated oxidative injury in the pathogenesis of some ILDs.[78] There have been no studies evaluating the effects of LTOT on pulmonary hemodynamics or RV dysfunction in patients with ILD-associated PH.

Pulmonary Disease-Specific Therapies

Therapies targeting the underlying pulmonary disease are routinely recommended for treatment of Group 3 disorders but these recommendations are not based on strong clinical evidence. Disease-specific therapies improve alveolar oxygenation, decrease V/Q mismatch, or limit the mechanical effects of hyperinflation on the pulmonary circulation.

Inhaled bronchodilators, anticholinergics, and corticosteroids remain the mainstay of therapy in obstructive lung diseases. These drugs, alone or in combination, have been shown to improve FEV_1 and reduce exacerbation frequency in COPD.[79,80] Short-acting β-agonists and inhaled anticholinergics modestly reduced PA pressures during exercise in patients with COPD but there was no change in the PVR.[81] Given the associated improvements in pulmonary artery occlusion pressure with these medications, PA pressure was probably reduced through improvements in lung mechanics. Oral theophylline has been associated with improved PA pressure, PVR, and cardiac index in patients with COPD[82] but these effects are strongly dependent on blood levels, even within the therapeutic range.[83] Theophylline is used infrequently in patients with COPD because of the narrow therapeutic window and because drug clearance be reduced in patients with diminished cardiac output.

Few effective disease-specific therapies are available for patients with ILD. These therapies are likely to have limited value in mitigating the associated PH, which usually develops in advanced disease when fibrotic remodeling is unlikely to respond to currently available therapies. There are limited data to suggest that corticosteroids may improve hemodynamics in diseases like sarcoidosis[54,84] and pulmonary Langerhans cell histiocytosis.[85] These hemodynamic improvements were not routinely associated with radiographic improvements and may be related to effects on the vasculitic components of these disorders. Idiopathic pulmonary fibrosis is poorly responsive to available therapies and current guidelines recommend against immunomodulatory pharmacotherapy for most patients with IPF.[86]

In obstructive sleep apnea, weight loss is recommended for all obese patients and is effective in reducing the frequency of apneic episodes.[87,88] In patients with OHS, surgically-induced weight loss has been associated with significant improvement in pulmonary hemodynamics.[89] Patients with mild to moderate OSA can be treated surgically with uvulopalatopharyngoplasty (UVPP), which has been associated with modest increase in RV ejection fraction.[90] In severe OSA, nasal continuous positive airway pressure (nCPAP) is the preferred treatment and directly improves hemodynamics. Patients with severe OSA treated with nCPAP for 4 months demonstrated reduced resting PA pressure and PVR; and exposure to acute hypoxia caused attenuated pulmonary vasoconstriction in nCPAP-treated patients when compared with pretreatment baselines.[91] Although multiple potential benefits can explain these findings (including reduction in nocturnal hypoxic episodes and improvement in cardiac function), the reduction in acute hypoxic pulmonary vasoreactivity suggests that nCPAP probably improves endothelial cell function.

Pulmonary Hypertension-Specific Therapies

Although therapies specifically designed to mitigate dysfunctional endothelial signaling and reduce pulmonary vascular tone have been used successfully to minimize the morbidity associated with pulmonary arterial hypertension, the data supporting use of these medications in PH and RV dysfunction associated with chronic lung disease are less compelling. The limited available data predominantly show acute improvements in cardio-pulmonary hemodynamics but fail to show longterm functional benefits. In several cases, these medications actually worsened hypoxemia by preventing hypoxic pulmonary vasoconstriction, and impaired RV function by reducing venous return. Currently, these therapies are not recommended for treatment of PH associated with chronic lung disease.[92]

Inhaled nitric oxide (NO) is a pulmonary vasodilator that has been successfully used in clinical trials to improve hemodynamics and exercise capacity in patients with COPD-associated pulmonary hypertension. COPD patients who inhaled NO in addition to supplemental oxygen, showed significant improvements in mean PA pressure, PVR, and cardiac output.[93] Inhaled NO improved V/Q matching and stabilized PaO_2 during exercise in patients with COPD-associated PH.[94] However, the need for continuous inhalation makes this therapy too cumbersome to be practical.

Sildenafil enhances the effects of NO on pulmonary vascular smooth muscle cells and causes pulmonary vasodilatation by inhibiting the enzyme phosphodiesterase-5 (PDE5). PDE5 is the predominant phosphodiesterase isoform in lung tissue and is responsible for catabolism of the NO second messenger cyclic guanosine monophosphate (cGMP). By inhibiting PDE5, sildenafil promotes accumulation of cGMP after NO stimulation, leading to smooth muscle cell relaxation and growth inhibition. COPD patients with pulmonary hypertension showed an acute reduction in resting and exercise-induced mean PA pressure and increased cardiac output during exercise after the administration of sildenafil.[95] Unfortunately, sildenafil was associated with a significant reduction in PaO_2 because of adverse effects on V/Q matching. The longterm benefits of sildenafil in COPD patients with PH have not been demonstrated. The limited available data regarding the potential efficacy of PDE5 inhibitors in ILD are conflicting. Whereas an initial open label trial of sildenafil in IPF patients with PH showed improvements in 6MWD after 12 weeks of therapy,[96] a later randomized clinical trial failed to replicate these findings.[97] Patients with severe IPF treated with sildenafil reported less dyspnea and had improved PaO_2 and D_LCO when compared with patients treated with placebo, although the potential effects of sildenafil on pulmonary hemodynamics were not reported.[97]

Endothelin 1 is produced by endothelial cells and has direct vasoconstrictor and mitogenic effects on vascular smooth muscle cells. The vasoconstrictive effects of endothelin are mediated by 2 receptors (ERA and ERB) on pulmonary arterial smooth muscle cells. Conversely, ERB is also functional on endothelial cells and stimulation mediates NO production and prostacyclin release, resulting in endothelial-mediated vasodilatation.

The endothelin receptor antagonists currently available, either target both receptors (bosentan), or selectively target ERA (sitaxsentan, ambrisentan). Bosentan has been evaluated in a randomized, controlled trial of PH patients with severe or very severe COPD.[98] The results were disappointing, because patients treated with 12 weeks of bosentan therapy showed no improvement in 6MWD or pulmonary hemodynamics. Bosentan-treated subjects had reduced PaO_2, widened alveolar-arterial oxygen gradient, and reported reduced quality of life when compared with subjects in the placebo arm.[98] The selective ERA antagonist ambrisentan did not improve 6MWD in COPD or ILD patients with PH in the ARIES-3 trial,[99] and a phase III study of ambristentan in IPF patients with PH was stopped early because of lack of clinical efficacy.[39]

Prostacyclin, produced by the endothelial cells, is a potent vasodilator that inhibits platelet aggregation and effectively prevents the release of growth factors from endothelial cells, platelets, and macrophages. In the United States, prostacyclin analogs are available for delivery via intravenous (epoprostenol and treprostinil), subcutaneous (treprostinil), and inhaled (iloprost) routes. Acutely, intravenous prostacyclin analogs have been shown to improve mean PA pressure, PVR, and cardiac output in patients with COPD-associated pulmonary hypertension.[100] Unfortunately, systemically administered prostacyclin analogs have been associated with worsened V/Q matching in patients with COPD, particularly those with acute respiratory failure,[101] and ILD patients with PH.[102] Intravenous prostacyclin analogs also carry a theoretical risk of precipitating pulmonary edema in some patients with ILD, because pulmonary veno-occlusive lesions have been described in several pulmonary disorders, including IPF, sarcoidosis, pulmonary Langerhans cell histiocytosis, and SSc-associated ILD.[39]

Prostacyclin analog administration through an inhaled route may mitigate the limiting issues with V/Q mismatch and hypoxemia. COPD patients with PH were recently shown to have improved V/Q matching, a reduced alveolar-arterial oxygen gradient, and longer 6MWD after acute treatment with inhaled iloprost.[103] Future studies that show sustained functional or hemodynamic effects with longer treatment courses would be encouraging.

Statins

Statins (3-hydroxy-3-methyl-glutaryl-CoA reductase inhibitors) represent an intriguing class of medications that may improve RV dysfunction associated with chronic lung disease. A recent randomized, placebo-controlled trial showed that COPD patients with PH, who were treated with pravastatin for 6 months demonstrated a significant increase in exercise capacity, improved estimated systolic PA pressure, and reduced dyspnea scores when compared with patients on placebo.[104] In a cross-sectional study of patients with severe COPD undergoing right heart catheterization for lung transplant evaluation, statin use was associated with a modest reduction in mean PA pressure and pulmonary artery occlusion pressure, although there was no difference in PVR.[105] The mechanism by which statins influence pulmonary hemodynamics remains unknown, although Lee and colleagues[104] showed that the use of statins was associated with reduced endothelin-1 production in COPD patients with PH. The multicenter ASA-STAT trial[106] that showed no improvement in 6MWD in patients with pulmonary arterial hypertension taking simvastatin for 6 months, suggested that the observed effects in COPD patients with PH may be associated with primary statin effects on the underlying lung disease or associated comorbidities.

Surgical Options

Surgical intervention is rarely warranted for the mild RV dysfunction associated with chronic lung disease. However, given the increased mortality associated with even mild PH in chronic lung disease (see later), associated PH is an indication for transplant listing based on the most recent guidelines.[107] In patients with PH associated with chronic lung disease, the decision between single and double lung transplantation is highly individualized, although both single and double lung transplantation have been shown to effectively reduce mean PA pressure in patients with chronic lung disease and there seems to be no difference in longterm survival.[108]

Lung volume reduction surgery (LVRS) was initially considered to be a potentially useful option to limit RV dysfunction in obstructive lung disease, because of the theoretical benefits of minimizing thoracic hyperinflation. Whereas LVRS was shown to improve respiratory mechanics and increase PaO$_2$, there was no improvement in hemodynamic indices in patients undergoing LVRS compared with those treated medically.[109] Therefore, despite theoretical benefits, no data support the routine referral for LVRS in patients with PH associated with chronic lung disease.

CLINICAL OUTCOMES

Whereas RV remodeling and hypertrophy are fairly common in chronic lung disease, RV failure is not.

Despite this, the development of PH is uniformly associated with increased mortality in patients with chronic lung disease. In COPD, modest increases in mean PA pressure (>20 mm Hg) have been correlated with reduced survival.[110] Mean PA pressure was shown to be highly predictive of longterm survival in COPD patients on LTOT, with only 36% of patients with PA pressure greater than 25 mm Hg surviving for 5 years compared with 62% of COPD patients with PA pressure less than 25 mm Hg.[111] Similarly, the development of pulmonary hypertension has been associated with reduced survival in ILD. In patients with advanced IPF complicated by PH there was 1-year mortality of 28%, whereas in patients with advanced IPF without PH there was 1-year mortality of 5.5%.[12] Modest increases in PA pressure are predictive of reduced longterm survival in IPF patients, as shown in **Fig. 2**. IPF patients with mean PA pressure greater than 17 mm Hg had a 5-year survival of only 16.7%, compared with IPF patients with mean PA pressure less than 17 mm Hg, who had 5-year survival of 62.2%.[11] In sarcoidosis, PH is an independent predictor of mortality[112] and the hazard ratio for death in patients with PH was estimated to be 10.4 when compared with patients without PH.[113] In patients with SSc-associated interstitial lung disease complicated by PH, there was a fivefold increased risk of death when compared with SSc patients with PAH, despite notoriously poor survival in this disorder.[56] Data regarding mortality

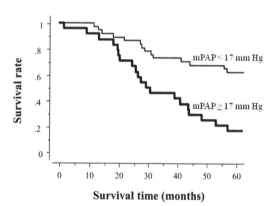

Fig. 2. Prognostic impact of mean pulmonary arterial pressure (mPAP) on survival in patients with idiopathic pulmonary fibrosis (IPF). Thin line represents IPF patients with normal mPAP (n = 37); thick line represents IPF patients with elevated mPAP (n = 24). (*Adapted from* Hamada K, Nagai S, Tanaka S, et al. Significance of pulmonary arterial pressure and diffusion capacity of the lung as prognosticator in patients with idiopathic pulmonary fibrosis. Chest 2007; 131(3):650–6; with permission.)

caused by PH in patients with sleep-disordered breathing are more challenging to interpret, primarily because of the frequent comorbidities in this group. Whereas the 1-, 3-, and 5-year survival estimates in OSA patients with mean PA pressure greater than 25 mm Hg (93%, 75%, and 43%, respectively) were reduced when compared with survival estimates in patients with OSA with normal PA pressures (100%, 90%, and 76%), only 31% of subjects with elevated mean PA pressure had normal pulmonary artery occlusion pressure.[114]

COMPLICATIONS AND CONCERNS

The primary complication associated with RV dysfunction in chronic lung disease is progression to RV failure. This is a rare complication in most circumstances but some clinical scenarios require special consideration. In COPD, acute exacerbations are associated with increased V/Q mismatch and reduced PaO_2.[115] It was noted that during acute exacerbations, some patients with COPD developed markedly increased RV end-diastolic pressures, potentially consistent with RV failure.[116] In this study, changes in RV end-diastolic pressure were associated with the development of peripheral edema, CO_2 retention, decreased arterial oxygen saturation, and increased mean PA pressure. RV contractility was reduced in a small cohort of COPD patients evaluated by right heart catheterization following the development of acute peripheral edema.[117] There is a subgroup of patients with COPD who appear to be at risk for development of more severe PH despite stable lung disease. This group accounted for 1.1% of all patients with COPD undergoing hemodynamic evaluation in one large retrospective analysis,[73] and has a unique clinical phenotype characterized by mild to moderate airways obstruction, severely reduced D_LCO, and severe hypoxemia. The incidence of RV failure in this subgroup is unknown. Patients with multiple chronic lung diseases, including overlap syndromes between COPD and OSA or ILD, may also be at increased risk for more severe RV dysfunction.

SUMMARY

Although the exact prevalence of RV dysfunction is unknown, sufficient evidence suggests that it is a common complication of chronic pulmonary disease. The pathophysiology is characterized by mildly increased PA pressures, RV hypertrophy, and preserved RV contractility and cardiac output. However, RV dysfunction can occasionally progress to RV failure during disease exacerbations

or when multiple cardio-pulmonary comorbidities are present. Patients with severe pulmonary hypertension that is out of proportion to the underlying lung disease should be screened for these comorbidities. The mechanism of RV dysfunction is associated primarily with hypoxic pulmonary vasoconstriction, pulmonary vascular remodeling, and disruption of pulmonary vascular beds caused by the underlying lung disease. Therefore, current recommendations support the use of LTOT and pulmonary disease-specific treatments, although evidence supporting improvements in RV function is limited. Therapies designed specifically to alter pulmonary vascular tone are currently not recommended for PH associated with chronic lung disease, because there are limited efficacy data and multiple reports of worsening hypoxemia. Some patients with severe pulmonary hypertension, associated only with chronic lung disease and out of proportion to the underlying pulmonary disease, should be considered for enrollment in clinical trials of these or other agents. For selected patients with severe parenchymal lung disease complicated by PH and RV dysfunction, lung transplantation should be an early consideration.

REFERENCES

1. Laennec RT. A treatise on diseases of the chest. London: T. and G. Underwood; 1821.
2. Chronic cor pulmonale: report of an expert committee. Circulation 1963;27:594–615.
3. Simonneau G, Robbins IM, Beghetti M, et al. Updated clinical classification of pulmonary hypertension. J Am Coll Cardiol 2009;54(Suppl 1): S43–54.
4. Ben Jrad I, Slimane ML, Boujnah MR, et al. Prognosis and treatment of chronic cor pulmonale. Tunis Med 1993;71(11):505–8 [in French].
5. Weitzenblum E, Chaouat A, Canuet M, et al. Pulmonary hypertension in chronic obstructive pulmonary disease and interstitial lung diseases. Semin Respir Crit Care Med 2009;30(4):458–70.
6. Hyduk A, Croft JB, Ayala C, et al. Pulmonary hypertension surveillance–United States, 1980-2002. MMWR Surveill Summ 2005;54(5):1–28.
7. Minai OA, Chaouat A, Adnot S. Pulmonary hypertension in COPD: epidemiology, significance, and management: pulmonary vascular disease: the global perspective. Chest 2010;137(Suppl 6): 39S–51S.
8. Scharf SM, Iqbal M, Keller C, et al. Hemodynamic characterization of patients with severe emphysema. Am J Respir Crit Care Med 2002;166(3): 314–22.

9. Badesch DB, Champion HC, Sanchez MA, et al. Diagnosis and assessment of pulmonary arterial hypertension. J Am Coll Cardiol 2009;54(Suppl 1): S55–66.

10. Han MK, McLaughlin VV, Criner GJ, et al. Pulmonary diseases and the heart. Circulation 2007; 116(25):2992–3005.

11. Hamada K, Nagai S, Tanaka S, et al. Significance of pulmonary arterial pressure and diffusion capacity of the lung as prognosticator in patients with idiopathic pulmonary fibrosis. Chest 2007; 131(3):650–6.

12. Lettieri CJ, Nathan SD, Barnett SD, et al. Prevalence and outcomes of pulmonary arterial hypertension in advanced idiopathic pulmonary fibrosis. Chest 2006;129(3):746–52.

13. Nathan SD, Shlobin OA, Ahmad S, et al. Pulmonary hypertension and pulmonary function testing in idiopathic pulmonary fibrosis. Chest 2007;131(3):657–63.

14. Sajkov D, McEvoy RD. Obstructive sleep apnea and pulmonary hypertension. Prog Cardiovasc Dis 2009;51(5):363–70.

15. Kessler R, Chaouat A, Schinkewitch P, et al. The obesity-hypoventilation syndrome revisited: a prospective study of 34 consecutive cases. Chest 2001;120(2):369–76.

16. Long term domiciliary oxygen therapy in chronic hypoxic cor pulmonale complicating chronic bronchitis and emphysema. Report of the Medical Research Council Working Party. Lancet 1981; 1(8222):681–6.

17. Bogaard HJ, Abe K, Vonk Noordegraaf A, et al. The right ventricle under pressure: cellular and molecular mechanisms of right-heart failure in pulmonary hypertension. Chest 2009;135(3):794–804.

18. Kayar SR, Banchero N. Myocardial capillarity in acclimation to hypoxia. Pflugers Arch 1985; 404(4):319–25.

19. Partovian C, Adnot S, Eddahibi S, et al. Heart and lung VEGF mRNA expression in rats with monocrotaline- or hypoxia-induced pulmonary hypertension. Am J Physiol 1998;275(6):H1948–56.

20. Vonk-Noordegraaf A, Marcus JT, Holverda S, et al. Early changes of cardiac structure and function in COPD patients with mild hypoxemia. Chest 2005; 127(6):1898–903.

21. Scott KW. A clinicopathological study of fatal chronic airways obstruction. Thorax 1976;31(6):693–701.

22. Shivkumar K, Ravi K, Henry JW, et al. Right ventricular dilatation, right ventricular wall thickening, and Doppler evidence of pulmonary hypertension in patients with a pure restrictive ventilatory impairment. Chest 1994;106(6):1649–53.

23. Bradley TD, Rutherford R, Grossman RF, et al. Role of daytime hypoxemia in the pathogenesis of right heart failure in the obstructive sleep apnea syndrome. Am Rev Respir Dis 1985;131(6):835–9.

24. Guidry UC, Mendes LA, Evans JC, et al. Echocardiographic features of the right heart in sleep-disordered breathing: the Framingham Heart Study. Am J Respir Crit Care Med 2001;164(6): 933–8.

25. Dursunoglu N, Dursunoglu D, Kilic M. Impact of obstructive sleep apnea on right ventricular global function: sleep apnea and myocardial performance index. Respiration 2005;72(3):278–84.

26. Vizza CD, Lynch JP, Ochoa LL, et al. Right and left ventricular dysfunction in patients with severe pulmonary disease. Chest 1998;113(3): 576–83.

27. Burghuber OC, Bergmann H. Right-ventricular contractility in chronic obstructive pulmonary disease: a combined radionuclide and hemodynamic study. Respiration 1988;53(1):1–12.

28. Biernacki W, Flenley DC, Muir AL, et al. Pulmonary hypertension and right ventricular function in patients with COPD. Chest 1988;94(6):1169–75.

29. Caso P, Galderisi M, Cicala S, et al. Association between myocardial right ventricular relaxation time and pulmonary arterial pressure in chronic obstructive lung disease: analysis by pulsed Doppler tissue imaging. J Am Soc Echocardiogr 2001;14(10):970–7.

30. Huez S, Retailleau K, Unger P, et al. Right and left ventricular adaptation to hypoxia: a tissue Doppler imaging study. Am J Physiol Heart Circ Physiol 2005;289(4):H1391–8.

31. Archer S, Michelakis E. The mechanism(s) of hypoxic pulmonary vasoconstriction: potassium channels, redox O(2) sensors, and controversies. News Physiol Sci 2002;17:131–7.

32. Enson Y, Giuntini C, Lewis ML, et al. The influence of hydrogen ion concentration and hypoxia on the pulmonary circulation. J Clin Invest 1964;43: 1146–62.

33. Timms RM, Khaja FU, Williams GW. Hemodynamic response to oxygen therapy in chronic obstructive pulmonary disease. Ann Intern Med 1985;102(1): 29–36.

34. Girgis RE, Mathai SC. Pulmonary hypertension associated with chronic respiratory disease. Clin Chest Med 2007;28(1):219–32.

35. Wilkinson M, Langhorne CA, Heath D, et al. A pathophysiological study of 10 cases of hypoxic cor pulmonale. Q J Med 1988;66(249):65–85.

36. Penaloza D, Arias-Stella J. The heart and pulmonary circulation at high altitudes: healthy highlanders and chronic mountain sickness. Circulation 2007;115(9):1132–46.

37. Matsuoka S, Washko GR, Yamashiro T, et al. Pulmonary hypertension and computed tomography measurement of small pulmonary vessels in severe emphysema. Am J Respir Crit Care Med 2010;181(3):218–25.

38. Falk JA, Martin UJ, Scharf S, et al. Lung elastic recoil does not correlate with pulmonary hemodynamics in severe emphysema. Chest 2007;132(5):1476–84.

39. Shlobin OA, Nathan SD. Pulmonary hypertension secondary to interstitial lung disease. Expert Rev Respir Med 2011;5(2):179–89.

40. Nathan SD, Noble PW, Tuder RM. Idiopathic pulmonary fibrosis and pulmonary hypertension: connecting the dots. Am J Respir Crit Care Med 2007;175(9):875–80.

41. Tillie-Leblond I, Marquette CH, Perez T, et al. Pulmonary embolism in patients with unexplained exacerbation of chronic obstructive pulmonary disease: prevalence and risk factors. Ann Intern Med 2006;144(6):390–6.

42. Rizkallah J, Man SF, Sin DD. Prevalence of pulmonary embolism in acute exacerbations of COPD: a systematic review and metaanalysis. Chest 2009;135(3):786–93.

43. Swigris JJ, Olson AL, Huie TJ, et al. Increased risk of pulmonary embolism among US decedents with sarcoidosis from 1988 to 2007. Chest 2011;140(5):1261–6.

44. Panos RJ, Mortenson RL, Niccoli SA, et al. Clinical deterioration in patients with idiopathic pulmonary fibrosis: causes and assessment. Am J Med 1990;88(4):396–404.

45. Fessler HE. Heart-lung interactions: applications in the critically ill. Eur Respir J 1997;10(1):226–37.

46. Watz H, Waschki B, Meyer T, et al. Decreasing cardiac chamber sizes and associated heart dysfunction in COPD: role of hyperinflation. Chest 2010;138(1):32–8.

47. Buda AJ, Pinsky MR, Ingels NB Jr, et al. Effect of intrathoracic pressure on left ventricular performance. N Engl J Med 1979;301(9):453–9.

48. Macnee W. Right heart function in COPD. Semin Respir Crit Care Med 2010;31(3):295–312.

49. Oswald-Mammosser M, Oswald T, Nyankiye E, et al. Non-invasive diagnosis of pulmonary hypertension in chronic obstructive pulmonary disease. Comparison of ECG, radiological measurements, echocardiography and myocardial scintigraphy. Eur J Respir Dis 1987;71(5):419–29.

50. Tan RT, Kuzo R, Goodman LR, et al. Utility of CT scan evaluation for predicting pulmonary hypertension in patients with parenchymal lung disease. Medical College of Wisconsin Lung Transplant Group. Chest 1998;113(5):1250–6.

51. Zisman DA, Karlamangla AS, Ross DJ, et al. High-resolution chest CT findings do not predict the presence of pulmonary hypertension in advanced idiopathic pulmonary fibrosis. Chest 2007;132(3):773–9.

52. Steen VD, Graham G, Conte C, et al. Isolated diffusing capacity reduction in systemic sclerosis. Arthritis Rheum 1992;35(7):765–70.

53. Nadrous HF, Pellikka PA, Krowka MJ, et al. Pulmonary hypertension in patients with idiopathic pulmonary fibrosis. Chest 2005;128(4):2393–9.

54. Nunes H, Humbert M, Capron F, et al. Pulmonary hypertension associated with sarcoidosis: mechanisms, haemodynamics and prognosis. Thorax 2006;61(1):68–74.

55. Gartman EJ, Blundin M, Klinger JR, et al. Initial risk assessment for pulmonary hypertension in patients with COPD. Lung 2012;190(1):83–9.

56. Mathai SC, Hummers LK, Champion HC, et al. Survival in pulmonary hypertension associated with the scleroderma spectrum of diseases: impact of interstitial lung disease. Arthritis Rheum 2009;60(2):569–77.

57. Steen V, Medsger TA Jr. Predictors of isolated pulmonary hypertension in patients with systemic sclerosis and limited cutaneous involvement. Arthritis Rheum 2003;48(2):516–22.

58. Leuchte HH, Neurohr C, Baumgartner R, et al. Brain natriuretic peptide and exercise capacity in lung fibrosis and pulmonary hypertension. Am J Respir Crit Care Med 2004;170(4):360–5.

59. Arena R, Guazzi M, Myers J, et al. Cardiopulmonary exercise testing in the assessment of pulmonary hypertension. Expert Rev Respir Med 2011;5(2):281–93.

60. Holverda S, Bogaard HJ, Groepenhoff H, et al. Cardiopulmonary exercise test characteristics in patients with chronic obstructive pulmonary disease and associated pulmonary hypertension. Respiration 2008;76(2):160–7.

61. Vonbank K, Funk GC, Marzluf B, et al. Abnormal pulmonary arterial pressure limits exercise capacity in patients with COPD. Wien Klin Wochenschr 2008;120(23–24):749–55.

62. Glaser S, Noga O, Koch B, et al. Impact of pulmonary hypertension on gas exchange and exercise capacity in patients with pulmonary fibrosis. Respir Med 2009;103(2):317–24.

63. Leuchte HH, Baumgartner RA, Nounou ME, et al. Brain natriuretic peptide is a prognostic parameter in chronic lung disease. Am J Respir Crit Care Med 2006;173(7):744–50.

64. Inoue Y, Kawayama T, Iwanaga T, et al. High plasma brain natriuretic peptide levels in stable COPD without pulmonary hypertension or cor pulmonale. Intern Med 2009;48(7):503–12.

65. Holverda S, Rietema H, Westerhof N, et al. Stroke volume increase to exercise in chronic obstructive pulmonary disease is limited by increased pulmonary artery pressure. Heart 2009;95(2):137–41.

66. Barr RG, Bluemke DA, Ahmed FS, et al. Percent emphysema, airflow obstruction, and impaired left ventricular filling. N Engl J Med 2010;362(3):217–27.

67. Gao Y, Du X, Liang L, et al. Evaluation of right ventricular function by 64-row CT in patients with chronic obstructive pulmonary disease and cor pulmonale. Eur J Radiol 2012;81(2):345–53.

68. Burgess MI, Bright-Thomas R. Usefulness of transcutaneous Doppler jugular venous echo to predict pulmonary hypertension in COPD patients. Eur Respir J 2002;19(2):382–3.

69. Arcasoy SM, Christie JD, Ferrari VA, et al. Echocardiographic assessment of pulmonary hypertension in patients with advanced lung disease. Am J Respir Crit Care Med 2003; 167(5):735–40.

70. Fisher MR, Criner GJ, Fishman AP, et al. Estimating pulmonary artery pressures by echocardiography in patients with emphysema. Eur Respir J 2007; 30(5):914–21.

71. Forfia PR, Fisher MR, Mathai SC, et al. Tricuspid annular displacement predicts survival in pulmonary hypertension. Am J Respir Crit Care Med 2006;174(9):1034–41.

72. Mertens LL, Friedberg MK. Imaging the right ventricle–current state of the art. Nat Rev Cardiol 2010;7(10):551–63.

73. Chaouat A, Bugnet AS, Kadaoui N, et al. Severe pulmonary hypertension and chronic obstructive pulmonary disease. Am J Respir Crit Care Med 2005;172(2):189–94.

74. Egan TM, Murray S, Bustami RT, et al. Development of the new lung allocation system in the United States. Am J Transplant 2006;6(5 Pt 2):1212–27.

75. Continuous or nocturnal oxygen therapy in hypoxemic chronic obstructive lung disease: a clinical trial. Nocturnal Oxygen Therapy Trial Group. Ann Intern Med 1980;93(3):391–8.

76. Zielinski J, Tobiasz M, Hawrylkiewicz I, et al. Effects of long-term oxygen therapy on pulmonary hemodynamics in COPD patients: a 6-year prospective study. Chest 1998;113(1): 65–70.

77. Crockett AJ, Cranston JM, Antic N. Domiciliary oxygen for interstitial lung disease. Cochrane Database Syst Rev 2001;3:CD002883.

78. Kliment CR, Oury TD. Oxidative stress, extracellular matrix targets, and idiopathic pulmonary fibrosis. Free Radic Biol Med 2010;49(5):707–17.

79. Calverley PM, Anderson JA, Celli B, et al. Salmeterol and fluticasone propionate and survival in chronic obstructive pulmonary disease. N Engl J Med 2007;356(8):775–89.

80. Tashkin DP, Celli B, Senn S, et al. A 4-year trial of tiotropium in chronic obstructive pulmonary disease. N Engl J Med 2008;359(15):1543–54.

81. Saito S, Miyamoto K, Nishimura M, et al. Effects of inhaled bronchodilators on pulmonary hemodynamics at rest and during exercise in patients with COPD. Chest 1999;115(2):376–82.

82. Matthay RA. Favorable cardiovascular effects of theophylline in COPD. Chest 1987;92(Suppl 1): 22S–6S.

83. Mols P, Huynh CH, Dechamps P, et al. Dose dependency of aminophylline effects on hemodynamic and ventricular function in patients with chronic obstructive pulmonary disease. Chest 1993;103(6):1725–31.

84. Gluskowski J, Hawrylkiewicz I, Zych D, et al. Effects of corticosteroid treatment on pulmonary haemodynamics in patients with sarcoidosis. Eur Respir J 1990;3(4):403–7.

85. Benyounes B, Crestani B, Couvelard A, et al. Steroid-responsive pulmonary hypertension in a patient with Langerhans' cell granulomatosis (histiocytosis X). Chest 1996;110(1):284–6.

86. Raghu G, Collard HR, Egan JJ, et al. An official ATS/ERS/JRS/ALAT statement: idiopathic pulmonary fibrosis: evidence-based guidelines for diagnosis and management. Am J Respir Crit Care Med 2011;183(6):788–824.

87. Grunstein RR, Stenlof K, Hedner JA, et al. Two year reduction in sleep apnea symptoms and associated diabetes incidence after weight loss in severe obesity. Sleep 2007;30(6):703–10.

88. Johansson K, Neovius M, Lagerros YT, et al. Effect of a very low energy diet on moderate and severe obstructive sleep apnoea in obese men: a randomised controlled trial. BMJ 2009;339:b4609.

89. Sugerman HJ, Baron PL, Fairman RP, et al. Hemodynamic dysfunction in obesity hypoventilation syndrome and the effects of treatment with surgically induced weight loss. Ann Surg 1988;207(5):604–13.

90. Zohar Y, Talmi YP, Frenkel H, et al. Cardiac function in obstructive sleep apnea patients following uvulopalatopharyngoplasty. Otolaryngol Head Neck Surg 1992;107(3):390–4.

91. Sajkov D, Wang T, Saunders NA, et al. Continuous positive airway pressure treatment improves pulmonary hemodynamics in patients with obstructive sleep apnea. Am J Respir Crit Care Med 2002; 165(2):152–8.

92. Hoeper MM, Barbera JA, Channick RN, et al. Diagnosis, assessment, and treatment of non-pulmonary arterial hypertension pulmonary hypertension. J Am Coll Cardiol 2009;54(Suppl 1): S85–96.

93. Vonbank K, Ziesche R, Higenbottam TW, et al. Controlled prospective randomised trial on the effects on pulmonary haemodynamics of the ambulatory long term use of nitric oxide and oxygen in patients with severe COPD. Thorax 2003;58(4):289–93.

94. Roger N, Barbera JA, Roca J, et al. Nitric oxide inhalation during exercise in chronic obstructive pulmonary disease. Am J Respir Crit Care Med 1997;156(3 Pt 1):800–6.

95. Blanco I, Gimeno E, Munoz PA, et al. Hemodynamic and gas exchange effects of sildenafil in patients with chronic obstructive pulmonary disease and pulmonary hypertension. Am J Respir Crit Care Med 2010;181(3):270–8.

96. Collard HR, Anstrom KJ, Schwarz MI, et al. Sildenafil improves walk distance in idiopathic pulmonary fibrosis. Chest 2007;131(3):897–9.

97. Zisman DA, Schwarz M, Anstrom KJ, et al. A controlled trial of sildenafil in advanced idiopathic pulmonary fibrosis. N Engl J Med 2010;363(7):620–8.

98. Stolz D, Rasch H, Linka A, et al. A randomised, controlled trial of bosentan in severe COPD. Eur Respir J 2008;32(3):619–28.

99. Badesch DB, Feldman J, Keogh A, et al. ARIES-3: Ambrisentan therapy in a diverse population of patients with pulmonary hypertension. Cardiovasc Ther 2012;30(2):93–9.

100. Naeije R, Melot C, Mols P, et al. Reduction in pulmonary hypertension by prostaglandin E1 in decompensated chronic obstructive pulmonary disease. Am Rev Respir Dis 1982;125(1):1–5.

101. Archer SL, Mike D, Crow J, et al. A placebo-controlled trial of prostacyclin in acute respiratory failure in COPD. Chest 1996;109(3):750–5.

102. Ghofrani HA, Wiedemann R, Rose F, et al. Sildenafil for treatment of lung fibrosis and pulmonary hypertension: a randomised controlled trial. Lancet 2002; 360(9337):895–900.

103. Dernaika TA, Beavin M, Kinasewitz GT. Iloprost improves gas exchange and exercise tolerance in patients with pulmonary hypertension and chronic obstructive pulmonary disease. Respiration 2010; 79(5):377–82.

104. Lee TM, Chen CC, Shen HN, et al. Effects of pravastatin on functional capacity in patients with chronic obstructive pulmonary disease and pulmonary hypertension. Clin Sci (Lond) 2009;116(6): 497–505.

105. Reed RM, Iacono A, DeFilippis A, et al. Statin therapy is associated with decreased pulmonary vascular pressures in severe COPD. COPD 2011; 8(2):96–102.

106. Kawut SM, Bagiella E, Lederer DJ, et al. Randomized clinical trial of aspirin and simvastatin for pulmonary arterial hypertension: ASA-STAT. Circulation 2011;123(25):2985–93.

107. Orens JB, Estenne M, Arcasoy S, et al. International guidelines for the selection of lung transplant candidates: 2006 update–a consensus report from the Pulmonary Scientific Council of the International Society for Heart and Lung Transplantation. J Heart Lung Transplant 2006;25(7):745–55.

108. Fitton TP, Kosowski TR, Barreiro CJ, et al. Impact of secondary pulmonary hypertension on lung transplant outcome. J Heart Lung Transplant 2005; 24(9):1254–9.

109. Criner GJ, Scharf SM, Falk JA, et al. Effect of lung volume reduction surgery on resting pulmonary hemodynamics in severe emphysema. Am J Respir Crit Care Med 2007;176(3):253–60.

110. Weitzenblum E, Hirth C, Ducolone A, et al. Prognostic value of pulmonary artery pressure in chronic obstructive pulmonary disease. Thorax 1981;36(10):752–8.

111. Oswald-Mammosser M, Weitzenblum E, Quoix E, et al. Prognostic factors in COPD patients receiving long-term oxygen therapy. Importance of pulmonary artery pressure. Chest 1995;107(5):1193–8.

112. Shorr AF, Davies DB, Nathan SD. Predicting mortality in patients with sarcoidosis awaiting lung transplantation. Chest 2003;124(3):922–8.

113. Baughman RP, Engel PJ, Taylor L, et al. Survival in sarcoidosis-associated pulmonary hypertension: the importance of hemodynamic evaluation. Chest 2010;138(5):1078–85.

114. Minai OA, Ricaurte B, Kaw R, et al. Frequency and impact of pulmonary hypertension in patients with obstructive sleep apnea syndrome. Am J Cardiol 2009;104(9):1300–6.

115. Barbera JA, Roca J, Ferrer A, et al. Mechanisms of worsening gas exchange during acute exacerbations of chronic obstructive pulmonary disease. Eur Respir J 1997;10(6):1285–91.

116. Weitzenblum E, Apprill M, Oswald M, et al. Pulmonary hemodynamics in patients with chronic obstructive pulmonary disease before and during an episode of peripheral edema. Chest 1994; 105(5):1377–82.

117. MacNee W, Wathen CG, Flenley DC, et al. The effects of controlled oxygen therapy on ventricular function in patients with stable and decompensated cor pulmonale. Am Rev Respir Dis 1988; 137(6):1289–95.

Right Ventricular Adaptation and Maladaptation in Chronic Pulmonary Arterial Hypertension

Stuart Rich, MD

KEYWORDS

- Right ventricle • Pulmonary hypertension • Heart failure
- Adaptation • Maladaptation

The right ventricle (RV) is not well suited to chronic pressure overload and often fails to adequately compensate. Mechanisms that allow the RV to respond to acute pressure overload often become maladaptive and contribute to its failure, including the effects of pulmonary hypertension (PH) on RV myocardial perfusion, the influence of interventricular dependence on RV function, and metabolic shifts in the RV myocardium from fatty acid to glycolysis.

CHARACTERISTICS OF THE NORMAL RIGHT VENTRICLE

The fetal right ventricle (RV) is a thick-walled chamber that ejects blood at relatively high pressures into a high-resistance pulmonary vascular bed. In humans, RV and left ventricle (LV) wall thickness increase in parallel between 12 weeks and term, with both chambers being roughly equal in thickness at birth. At birth, the pulmonary circulation remodels, becomes a low-pressure-low resistance circuit, and blood no longer bypasses the lung following closure of the foramen ovale and ductus arteriosus.[1] The RV ejects blood directly into the pulmonary artery and, as the pulmonary vascular resistance falls, right ventricular hypertrophy (RVH) regresses leaving the adult pattern of a thin-walled RV that is one third the thickness of the adult LV. Although the molecular signals that initiate this process remain uncertain, it has been suggested that inactivation of fetal genes responsible for hypertrophy of the RV play a role in normal adaptation.

The crescent-shaped RV has a distinct geometry from the cone-shaped LV, and the mechanism of contraction of the RV is quite different from the LV.[2] The superficial RV myocardial fibers are arrayed circumferentially and are in continuity with the LV fibers, explaining the motion of the RV free wall toward the interventricular septum in systole (Fig. 1).[3] A deeper layer of vertically arrayed RV fibers accounts for systolic shortening of the RV. RV contraction begins at the inflow region and progresses toward the outflow tract (likened to a bellows). In distinction, the LV contracts in a squeezing motion (likened to wringing a towel) from the LV apex to the outflow tract (Fig. 2). These differing mechanics allow the RV to rapidly adapt to volume overload conditions and the LV to pressure overload conditions, which are part of normal human physiology. The RV ejection fraction is slightly lower than the LV ejection fraction, but the slightly larger RV volume ensures a virtually identical cardiac output. In normal adults, studied using MRI, the RV ejection fraction is 61.6% ± 6.3% versus LV ejection fraction 64.8% ± 5.4%.[4]

Department of Medicine, Section of Cardiology, University of Chicago, 5841 South Maryland Avenue, MC 5403; Suite L 08, Chicago, IL 60637, USA
E-mail address: srich@medicine.bsd.uchicago.edu

Cardiol Clin 30 (2012) 257–269
doi:10.1016/j.ccl.2012.03.004

cardiology.theclinics.com

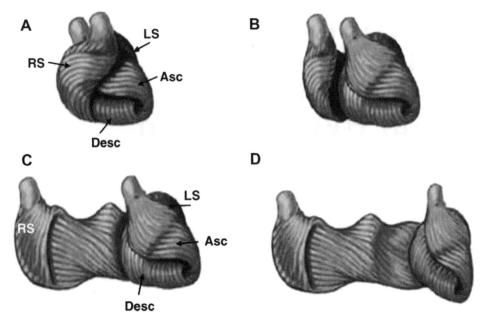

Fig. 1. Fiber orientation of the LVs and RVs and septum. In this heart model, the intact ventricle (*A*) is unfolded by the detachment of the pulmonary artery to unfold the basal segment (*B*). As it unfolds, note the obliquely oriented descending (Desc) and ascending (Asc) segments of the septum. With further unfolding of the RV from the left ventricular segment of the basal loop (*C*), the transverse fiber orientation of the RV free wall becomes apparent. As the heart becomes completely unfolded (*D*) note the obliquely oriented fibers within the descending and ascending segments of the apical loop that is responsible for septal motion. (*Adapted from* Saleh S, Liakopoulos OJ, Buckberg GD. The septal motor of biventricular function. Eur J Cardiothorac Surg 2006;29:S126–38; with permission.)

Right Ventricular Response to Exercise and Volume Overload

In response to exercise, where venous return to the right atrium can markedly increase, the RV can handle large volumes easily. Studies in normal subjects indicate that cardiac output increases with exercise largely because of an increase in RV stroke volume with end-diastolic volume unchanged.[5] The low-resistance pulmonary vasculature is able to accommodate the increased flow without an increase in pressure.

The highly compliant RV also has the ability to adapt to volume overload states from cardiac diseases. For example, in otherwise healthy individuals, removal of the tricuspid valve from endocarditis causes severe tricuspid regurgitation but generally leaves the patient able to function normally. In patients with atrial septal defects, who can have resting left-to-right shunts of greater than 4:1 with normal exercise capacity, the RV can function normally for decades.[6] Studies suggest, however, that chronic right ventricular volume overload eventually leads to high-output RV failure. For example, the presence of a flail tricuspid valve is associated with decreased survival and a higher incidence of symptomatic heart failure and atrial

fibrillation. Large, uncorrected atrial septal defects eventually cause progressive dyspnea with effort and RV failure.

Effects of PH on the RV

In the early stages of PH, RVH is mostly an adaptive response (compensated state). As the disease progresses, the RV dilates and RV failure eventually occurs (maladaptive right ventricular remodeling). The compensatory phase during the progressive increasing afterload is shorter in the RV compared with the LV and is consistent with the increased mortality observed in patients with PH compared with patients with systemic hypertension. The same is true with acute increases in the afterload. Cardiovascular collapse is common with massive pulmonary embolism but extremely rare in patients with a systemic hypertensive emergency. The reason for the increased vulnerability of the RV remains unclear.[7] An intriguing hypothesis involves the loss of the "protective" molecular, metabolic, and structural phenotype of the fetal RV, which extends into the adult life only in patients with congenital heart disease in whom the transition to the adult RV never occurs.[8] Thus, when the transition to the adult phenotype

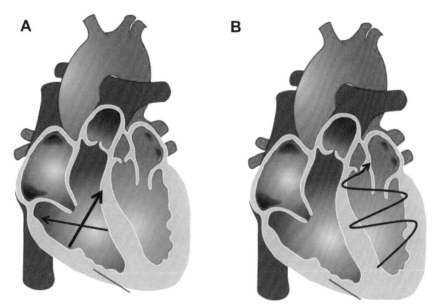

Fig. 2. Contrasting mechanisms of ventricular contraction. The RV is morphologically unique from the LV. It has a crescent-like shape and contracts with a peristaltic bellows-like action from apex to base. (*A*) The RV can accommodate large variations in venous return while maintaining a normal cardiac output. The bellows-like contraction results in a high ratio of RV volume change to RV free wall surface area change, which allows it to eject a large volume of blood with little alteration in RV wall stretch. The relatively flat relationship between the right ventricular surface area and volume limits the use of the Frank-Starling mechanism to increase the strike volume. The LV has a spherical shape with a distinctly different multiplanar action of contraction that is more like the wringing of a towel. (*B*) The helical nature of the myocardial bands allows for a twisting motion to eject and reciprocal untwisting to rapidly fill. The twisting action tends to initiate from the apex and progresses toward the base allowing for forceful ejection of blood against high resistance.

does occur, the RV becomes more vulnerable to failure in the presence of increased afterload due to the inability to switch back to the fetal program. The myocardial hypertrophy program has been elucidated (**Fig. 3**). A recent study demonstrated that genes may also be differentially regulated in the pressure-overloaded RV as compared with the pressure-overloaded LV.[9] The differential expression of genes in the right heart and left heart is not surprising in view of the different embryologic origin of the RV and LV and their different physiologic environments.[10]

Changes in Right Ventricular Size, Shape, and the Influence of Interventricular Dependence

In conditions in which RV systolic pressure or pulmonary vascular resistance is elevated, or when LV function is impaired, RV function becomes the major determinant of functional capacity and prognosis. Chronic pressure overload stimulates RV hypertrophy in an attempt to compensate for the increased afterload and maintain cardiac output without increasing wall stress.[11] However, not all pressure overloads are equivalent. When RV systolic pressure is increased from birth, the RV

develops characteristic concentric hypertrophy with preserved function. The classic example is pulmonic stenosis, in which the RV is often able to generate more than four times the normal RV systolic pressure for many years. In the adult with chronic pulmonic stenosis, the RV free wall and septum are hypertrophied, with RV volume maintained or slightly increased. Additionally, the septum retains its normal contour in continuity with the LV. It is possible that the persistent expression of fetal genes responsible for hypertrophy of the RV plays a role (**Fig. 4**).

Acquired RV pressure overload in adults, such as the result of pulmonary vascular diseases, produces adaptive and maladaptive RV responses, a qualitative differentiation based on the better preserved functional state and longer time to development of RV failure in those with adaptive RVH.[12] There are many factors that determine whether RVH will be well tolerated, such as the degree of autonomic activation, fibrosis, ischemia, and metabolic changes. The RV dilates to compensate for the reduced ejection fraction to maintain stroke volume.[13] The interventricular septum changes shape, and flattens or reverses its curvature. As the RV dilates, the tricuspid valve becomes

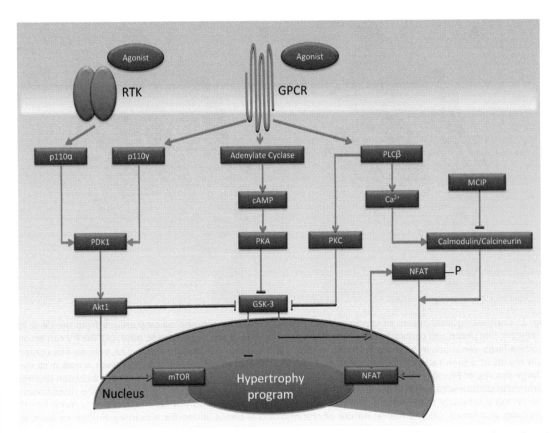

Fig. 3. Molecular pathways attributable to the hypertrophy program. G protein-coupled receptors (GPCRs) and receptor tyrosine kinase (RTK) signaling are involved in the myocardial hypertrophic response. On binding of ligands such as ATII and ET-1 to their G protein-coupled receptor, phospholipase C (PLCβ) is activated, which is followed by an increase in intracellular calcium (Ca2+) and protein kinase C (PKC) activation. This ultimately leads to dephosphorylation of the nuclear factor of activated T-cell (NFAT) transcription factor by calcineurin. Dephosphorylated nuclear factor of activated T cell translocates into the nucleus where it activates transcription in cooperation with other transcription factors. Dephosphorylation of nuclear factor of activated T cell by calcineurin is inhibited by glycogen synthase kinase-3 (GSK-3). After binding of catecholamines to the β-adrenergic receptor, adenylate cyclase is activated, cyclic adenosine monophosphate (cAMP) is produced, and protein kinase A (PKA) is activated. Phosphatidylinositol-3 kinase phosphorylates the membrane phospholipid phosphatidylinositol-4,5-biphosphate, which leads to the formation of phosphatylinositol-3,4,5-triphosphate (phosphatidylinositol-3 kinase) and recruitment of the protein kinase Akt1 to the cell membrane. Akt1 induces antiapoptotic and prohypertrophic responses by releasing transcription factors from tonic inhibition by glycogen synthase kinase-3 (GSK-3) and by activating mammalian target of rapamycin (mTOR). Binding of ATII, catecholamines, and ET-1 to their G protein-coupled receptor is associated with a similar pathway, involving Akt1 and another phosphatidylinositol-3 kinase subtype (p110γ). (*Adapted from* Bogaard HJ, Abe K, Vonk Noordegraaf A, et al. The RV under pressure. cellular and molecular mechanisms of right-heart failure in pulmonary hypertension. Chest 2009;134:794–4; with permission.)

incompetent and adds the additional burden of volume overload to the pressure-loaded RV. The RV also loses its normal diastolic compliance with right atrial pressure and RV end diastolic pressure rising, a powerful marker of survival.[14]

The importance of the septum versus the RV free wall has been highlighted. Studies have shown that the interventricular septum provides an important contribution to ventricular interaction and is important in the coupling of LV and RV systolic functions. It has been suggested that septal position may determine the magnitude of the LV-RV interaction, and that the correct angulation of the RV free wall and septal fibers are essential.[3] As a result, it seems necessary to maintain left ventricular pressure work to maximize right ventricular function. Clinical settings where this becomes apparent include the use of vasodilators that affect only the systemic circulation and in the use of mechanical support of the failing LV, which can often cause a significant worsening of RV function while simultaneously improving LV

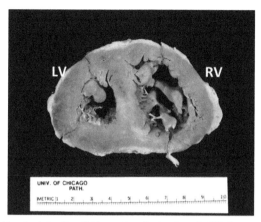

Fig. 4. Adaptive RV hypertrophy to chronic PH. A cross section of a postmortem heart of a patient that died with chronic severe PH that was well compensated is demonstrated. Notice the markedly increased wall thickness of the RV that is comparable to the LV. Additionally, the RV has not dilated. These characteristic changes allow the RV to adapt to a chronic high pressure state.

function.[15] Though not appreciated clinically, systemic hypotension can actually worsen RV function in patients with PH who are in severe right heart failure.

The mechanisms of interdependence are better understood by use of new imaging techniques. The classical echocardiographic appearance of severe PH is one of a markedly dilated RV and a small LV. It has been debated whether the mechanism of the small LV is compression that is contributing to the increased LV end diastolic pressure or underfilling because of the RV failure. Bernheim described the interdependence between the RV and LV, hypothesizing that the geometric changes from progressive LV enlargement and hypertrophy could directly compress the RV and thereby reduce RV filling. This "Bernheim effect" provided an explanation for the elevated central venous pressure and peripheral edema in cases of LV failure. The "reverse" Bernheim phenomenon (ie, enlargement of the RV leading to compression and underfilling of the LV) has been described in animals and humans with PH and RV failure.[16] Several echocardiographic studies have shown a high incidence of decreased early LV filling in patients with PH and RV enlargement. The LV appears distorted and compressed in the setting of severe RV pressure overload, and the interventricular septum seems to function more as part of the RV than the LV. Typically, there is reversal of the E/A wave transmitral flow pattern, a lower stroke volume index, and a lower cardiac index in PH versus control patients.

On the other hand, underfilling of the left heart is also a rational explanation for the observed physiology. Using MRI, patients with idiopathic pulmonary arterial hypertension (IPAH) had a reduction in LV peak filling rate and LV stroke volume as compared with control patients. Investigators also found that leftward curvature of the interventricular septum correlated with LV filling rate and concluded that direct ventricular interaction impairs left ventricular filling in PH.[16] A study in patients with chronic thromboembolic PH preoperatively and postoperatively also observed this phenomenon.[17] Preoperatively, the interventricular septum was not hypertrophied and its thickness matched that of the LV posterior wall. Postoperatively, the dramatic increases in transmitral E wave and pulmonary venous flow velocities after pulmonary thromboendarterectomy were consistent with a marked improvement in LV preload. The rapid normalization of the E/A wave ratio after pulmonary thromboendarterectomy and the presence of normal preoperative interventricular septal thickness by echo would also argue against any significant lingering effects from septal hypertrophy. Finally, the coexistence of an E/A wave transmitral filling pattern and an essentially normal early mitral annular velocity before pulmonary thromboendarterectomy is perhaps the most persuasive evidence of LV underfilling with relatively preserved diastolic function.

The Role of Ischemia on RV Function in PH

Adult patients with PH and RV failure often present with clinical features of myocardial ischemia. They experience angina-like chest pain, have elevated brain natriuretic peptide levels, and frequently have low levels of troponin release, which indicates a poor prognosis.[18] Normal physiology shows that the right coronary artery delivers blood to the RV continuously in systole and diastole. This is in distinction from left coronary artery flow, which delivers blood primarily in diastole. Resting right coronary blood flow is lower than left coronary blood flow, which is consistent with the lesser work of the RV. At rest, the LV extracts 75% of the oxygen delivered by coronary blood flow, whereas right ventricular oxygen extraction is only 50%.[19]

RV systolic perfusion is sensitive to elevated RV systolic pressure because RV hypertension attenuates the driving gradient for coronary perfusion during systole (aortic-RV systolic pressure). Thus, in PH, RV stroke work is markedly increased while right coronary perfusion is significantly reduced (**Fig. 5**).[20] Although the prevailing wisdom that decreased right coronary artery perfusion in

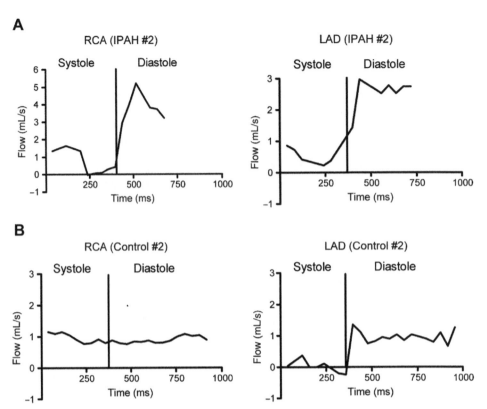

Fig. 5. Changes in RV myocardial blood flow in PH. Coronary artery blood flow as measured with cardiac MRI is shown. Patient (*A*) with chronic PH reveals predominant diastolic coronary artery blood flow in the right coronary artery and the left anterior descending coronary artery. Patient (*B*) is a normal patient that illustrates the continuous right coronary artery flow to a normal RV compared with the predominant diastolic coronary blood flow in the normal LV. LAD, left anterior descending; RCA, right coronary artery. (*From* van Wolferen SA, Marcus TJ, Westerhof N, et al. Right coronary artery flow impairment in patients with pulmonary hypertension. Eur Heart J 2008;29:120–7; with permission.)

systole as a result of elevated RV systolic pressure is the main cause of RV ischemia, this does not fully explain the disconnect between pulmonary artery pressure and prognosis. Although a severe reduction in coronary perfusion pressure can reduce RV function, RV contractile function remains constant until perfusion pressures fall below 50 mm Hg, which occurs only when patients become markedly hypotensive (**Fig. 6**).[20]

It is increasingly recognized that impairment of coronary perfusion pressure is not the only cause of ischemia. Rather, ischemia in RVH may reflect capillary rarefaction (ie, attenuation of small vessel density in the RV myocardium) that has been previously studied in left ventricular hypertrophy.[21] Rats with RVH caused by pulmonary artery banding have longer survival and better exercise tolerance than rats with a similar level of PH generated by the injection of monocrotaline or from the combination of a vascular endothelial growth factor receptor antagonist plus chronic hypoxia (**Fig. 7**). Notably, the latter two models produce

pulmonary vascular endothelial cell injury, which would support a potential role for molecular signaling from the pulmonary circulation because of endothelial damage or dysfunction, which affects the RV circulation itself. If there is significant microvascular disease in the hypertrophied RV in humans, it might be reasonable to treat RV failure by anti-ischemic agents. Conversely, if RV failure were initiated primarily by a drop in coronary perfusion pressure then current strategies, such as infusion of phenylephrine to increase the aortic-RV pressure gradient that drives coronary perfusion, might be a rational approach.

Changes in Cellular Metabolism with RVH

RV dysfunction may represent a form of myocardial hibernation (defined as reduced RV function due to chronic reduction in RV perfusion in the presence of viable myocardium).[22] Glycolysis and glucose oxidation are the major sources of ATP production in the fetal heart and the fetus is exposed to low

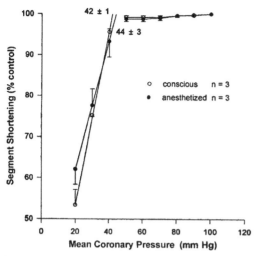

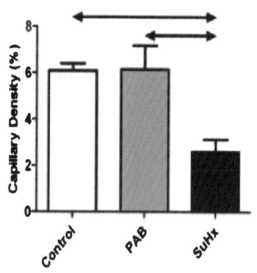

Fig. 6. Reduced coronary artery driving pressure can cause sudden cardiac decompensation. The mean coronary driving pressure (x axis) is shown along with right ventricular contractility (y axis) as measured by myocardial segment shortening in normal animals. Note how contractility falls dramatically when a critical point is reached in the coronary driving pressure as opposed to a gradual reduction in contractility proportional to the reduction in coronary blood flow. This physiology suggests that it is important to maintain a critical systolic blood pressure in patients presenting with acute right heart failure from chronic PH. (*From* Bian A, Williams AG Jr, Gwirtz PA, et al. Right coronary autoregulation in conscious chronically instrumented dogs. Am J Physiol Heart Circ Physiol 1998;275:H161–75; with permission.)

Fig. 7. Myocardial capillary density in animal models of PH. Myocardial capillary density is plotted in normal control animals, animals with right ventricular hypertension from pulmonary artery banding (PAB), and animals with PH from the combination of hypoxia and vascular endothelial growth factor receptor blockade model (SuHx). In the latter model, there is a significant reduction in capillary density of the right ventricular myocardium. This would suggest that there is molecular signaling between the pulmonary vasculature and the myocardial vasculature, which may result in RV ischemia. (*Adapted from* Bogaard HJ, Natarajan R, Henderson SC, et al. Chronic pulmonary artery pressure elevation is insufficient to explain right heart failure. Circulation 2009;120:1951–60; with permission.)

circulating fatty acid levels. However, in the adult, fatty acid oxidation becomes the predominant energy source (60%–90%). In contrast to the normal RV, which can vary its substrate use from fatty acids to glucose as needed, RVH is associated with a persistent reliance on glucose metabolism. Recent studies in rodent models suggest that in RVH the metabolic fate of glucose is altered because mitochondrial metabolism is actively (and reversibly) suppressed in the hypertrophied RV.[23] Thus, the primary fuel source becomes glycolysis as opposed to the fatty acid oxidation (**Fig. 8**).

At first, this seems paradoxic, because oxidative phosphorylation in the mitochondria produces much more ATP compared with glycolysis. However, it is possible that, in the presence of increased afterload, the myocardium suppresses mitochondrial-dependent apoptosis, in exchange for suboptimal contractility. In a study with animal models of PH, activating glucose oxidation using the phosphodiesterase (PDE) kinase (PDK) inhibitor dichloroacetate improved RV function while regressing RVH, which suggests that the RV can

be resuscitated metabolically.[24] This is consistent with a small series of PH patients studied with PET in which treatment with prostacyclin resulted in a shift back to fatty acid metabolism.[22] In a recent case report there was evidence of greater glycolysis and upregulation of PDK in the RV of a patient with maladaptive RVH and short survival than was seen in a patient with adaptive RVH and long survival (**Fig. 9**).[25] Thus, a therapeutic strategy of enhancing glucose oxidation, inhibiting ischemia, and avoiding inotropes to treat RV failure in PH patients merits investigation.[26]

The Response of the RV to Treatments of PH

Management of patients with acute and chronic RV failure is more empiric than the management of patients with left heart failure. Management of RV failure should always take into account the cause and setting in which the RV failure occurs. As in left heart failure, specific treatment goals include optimization of preload, afterload, and contractility, as well as maintenance of sinus rhythm and

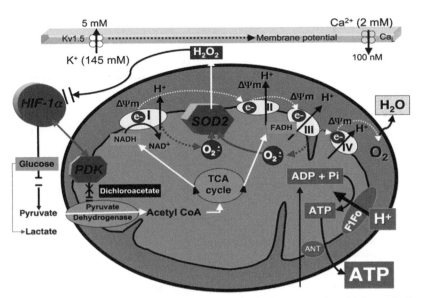

Fig. 8. Pathways for the metabolic shifts in RV myocardial metabolism. Mitochondrial metabolism in PAH. In aerobic metabolism, PDK is inactive, PDH is active, and electron donors (mitochondrial NADH and FADH) produced by the tricarboxylic acid cycle (TCA or Krebs cycle) pass electrons down a redox-potential gradient in the electron transport chain to molecular O_2. This electron flux powers H+ ion extrusion, which creates the proton-motive force responsible for creating the negative membrane potential ($\Delta\Psi m$) of mitochondria and powering F1Fo ATP synthase. Side reactions between semiquinones and molecular O_2, which account for $\approx$3% of net electron flux, create superoxide anion in proportion to po2. Superoxide dismutase (SOD2) rapidly converts superoxide anion (produced at complexes I and III) to H2O2, which serves as a redox messenger signaling "normoxia." In hypoxia (and PAH and cancer), there is activation of HIF-1α and PDK, which inhibits PDH, shifting metabolism toward glycolysis. Acetyl CoA indicates acetyl-coenzyme A. The upregulation of HIF-1α appears to be a major upstream transcription factor in the clinical development of PH. CoA, coenzyme A; FADH, flavin adenine dinucleotide; Glut1, glucose transporter 1; HIF-1a, hypoxia inducible factor-1 alpha; PAH, pulmonary arterial hypertension; PDH, pyruvate dehydrogenase; PDK, Pyruvate dehydrogenase kinase; PDK4, pyruvate dehydrogenase kinase, isozyme 4; TCA, trichloroacetic acid. (*Adapted from* Archer SL, Gomberg-Maitland M, Maitland M, et al. Mitochondrial metabolism, redox signaling, and fusion: a mitochondria-ROS-HIF-1alpha-Kv1.5 O2-sensing pathway at the intersection of pulmonary hypertension and cancer. Am J Physiol Heart Circ Physiol 2008; 294:H570–8; with permission.)

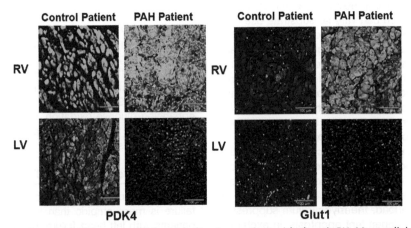

Fig. 9. Demonstration of a shift in myocardial metabolism in a patient with chronic PH. Myocardial stains for PDK 4 and Glut 1 in postmortem hearts from two patients, a control (normal) patient and a patient with PH, are shown. There is more intense staining in the RV of the patient compared with the LV, whereas the intensity of staining is comparable in both ventricles in the control patient. Both PDK4 and Glut1 are biochemical markers of glycolysis and confirm the metabolic shift away from a fatty acid substrate to glycolysis that occurs in the RV of patients with PH.

atrioventricular synchrony. Whether the use of diuretics and inotropic treatments in RV failure should follow similar practices to their use in LV failure is unknown. Additionally, the efficacy of drugs that counteract the renin-angiotensin system and the use of beta blockers in chronic RV failure have never been tested. The only classes of drugs for which clinical outcomes in chronic PH are known are the calcium channel blockers (CCB), endothelin receptor antagonists (ERA), PDE type 5 inhibitors (PDE5I), and prostacyclins.

CCBs

This class of drugs for a subset of PH patients has changed the treatment paradigm of PH. The initial experience demonstrated that high doses of nifedipine (Procardia) or diltiazem (Cardizem) could lower pressure and resistance in the pulmonary vasculature in select patients with IPAH.[27] With a fall in the pulmonary artery pressure (PAP), cardiac output increased, with no change in the systemic blood pressure. Patients most likely to respond to high doses of CCBs can be identified by hemodynamic testing with short-acting vasodilators at the time of the initial evaluation. Inhaled nitric oxide, intravenous epoprostenol, or intravenous adenosine can identify patients who acutely lower their PAP in response to vasodilators. It has been reported that 10% to 20% of patients with IPAH are vasoreactive. This response can be maintained in some patients for more than 15 years.[28] CCBs likely provide benefit solely through vasodilatation, as represented by the fall in PAP, because they have various degrees of negative inotropic effects. The increase in cardiac output that results is due to pressure unloading of the RV.

It is possible that these patients represent a subset of patients whose PH has been triggered by increased calcium in pulmonary artery smooth muscle cells due to abnormalities in the potassium channel.[29,30] The high doses of CCBs necessary to achieve the maximum beneficial effect in responders may be related to impaired absorption or to an increased requirement of calcium in the pulmonary vascular bed. The duration of the benefit in many of these patients seems to be indefinite. It is unknown whether the response to CCBs identifies two subsets of patients with IPAH, different stages of IPAH, or a combination. However, these patients seem to have less advanced disease as evidenced by a larger proportion of New York Heart Association functional class II patients and less severe hemodynamic parameters. No other clinical characteristics or baseline hemodynamic features allow one to predict those with or without a sustained response. This experience underscores that RV function will return to normal in patients with PH whose pulmonary artery pressure is markedly lowered.

ERAs

Endothelin-1 (ET-1) contributes to the pathophysiology of cardiac hypertrophy and failure. ET-1 exerts inotropic effects in human myocardium through endothelin type A (ETA) receptor–mediated increases in myofibrillar calcium responsiveness.[31] In dilated cardiomyopathy, the functional effects of ET-1 are attenuated, but ETA receptor density and ET-1 peptide concentration are increased, indicating an activated local cardiac ET system and possibly a reduced postreceptor signaling efficiency. ET-1 contributes to the Frank-Starling response in severely hypertrophied rat hearts. However, the inotropic effect of ET-1 accounts for only 20% to 30% of the maximal beta-adrenergic receptor–mediated inotropic effect in nonfailing and failing myocardium.[32]

This may explain a possible mechanism for the adverse effects of the endothelin antagonists (bosentan [Tracleer]) observed in patients with left heart failure.[33] In randomized clinical trials involving patients with LV failure, the use of bosentan has been associated with worsening outcomes. Although a similar effect has not been consistently observed in patients with RV failure and PH, the common finding of lower extremity edema in these patients raises the possibility that it may have also negative inotropic clinical effects in some patients with PH.[34] Clinical trials with ERAs have not shown a significant fall in pulmonary artery pressure or a reversal of RV remodeling. Special care should be taken with the use of ERAs in severe RVH.

PDE5Is

Whereas the expression of PDE type 5 (PDE5) is minimal in the normal RV (in which it is only expressed in the smooth muscle cells of the coronary arteries), its expression is markedly upregulated in the hypertrophied RV in rat and humans.[35] It is possible that its upregulation is a feature of the stressed myocardium because it parallels the induction of brain natriuretic peptide expression in the hypertrophied myocardium. As a result, PDE5Is have been shown to target the failing RV. PDE5I is also induced in the remodeled pulmonary arteries in PH and has beneficial effects on right ventricular afterload by dilating and reversing the remodeled pulmonary arteries, with minimal effects on the systemic arteries (**Fig. 10**).[36]

Sildenafil (Revatio) is a PDE5I that was once thought to act solely on the pulmonary vasculature. However, sildenafil has been found to have a direct RV inotropic effect that occurs in RVH. Sildenafil exerts a milrinone-like effect due to inhibition of PDE5 and, thus, increases cyclic guanosine monophosphate (GMP) levels that, through a process of molecular cross talk, inhibit PDE type 3 (PDE3).[37]

The appearance of a selective RV target accounts in part for the ability of sildenafil to increase cardiac output in PH. In randomized clinical trials, the use of sildenafil in patients with PH has shown

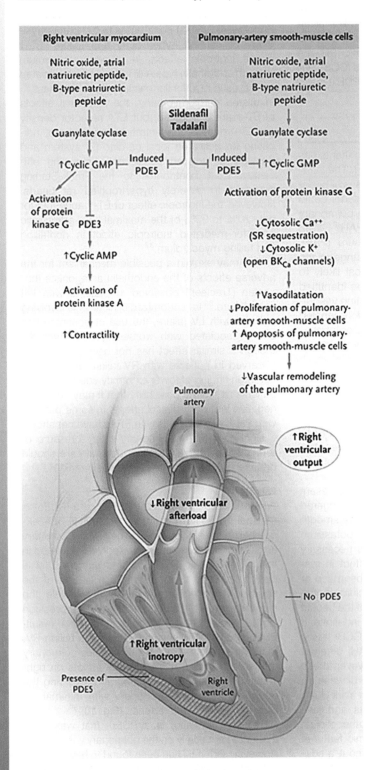

Fig. 10. Effects of PDE5I in pulmonary arterial hypertension. The combined effect of PDE5I on both the RV and the pulmonary artery (ie, increasing right ventricular inotropy and decreasing right ventricular afterload) may be more advantageous than drugs that affect only the pulmonary artery. Because PKG is much less abundant in the myocardium than in the vasculature, and because PKG activity is further decreased in RVH, the main effect of PDE5I is cyclic guanosine monophosphate–mediated inhibition of protein kinase A (a milrinone-like effect that increases right ventricular contractility). In contrast, in pulmonary-artery smooth-muscle cells, the effects of PDE5I are mediated by PKG and its multiple targets, leading to vasodilatation, reduced cell proliferation, and increased apoptosis. These combined effects lower the pulmonary vascular resistance. BK_{Ca} denotes the large conductance calcium-sensitive potassium channel, GMP, PDE3, PDE5, and SR sarcoplasmic reticulum. BK_{Ca}, the large conductance calcium-sensitive potassium channel; GMP, guanosine monophosphate; PDK, Pyruvate dehydrogenase kinase; SR, sarcoplasmic reticulum. (*Adapted from* Archer SL, Michelakis ED. Phosphodiesterase type 5 inhibitors for pulmonary arterial hypertension. N Engl J Med 2009;361:1864–71; with permission.)

dose-related increases in cardiac output over the duration of the trial.[38] In addition, it seems that the combination of sildenafil with intravenous prostacyclin produces synergistic increases in cardiac output.[39] Similar data does not exist for taldalafil (Adcirca), also approved for PH and, thus, it is unclear as to whether taldalafil and sildenafil are clinically equivalent.

Prostacyclins

Prostacyclin (Flolan) has been shown to cause an increase in contractility and cardiac output in animals and humans with both left and right heart failure.[40] It is believed that this is due to a direct effect on myocardial cyclic AMP. In patients with PH, cardiac output will predictably increase as the dose of prostacyclin is also increased.[41] It is particularly distinctive that these patients do not seem to develop ventricular arrhythmias or fibrillation while on chronic prostacyclin therapy in spite of its apparent inotropic effects as occurs in patients with chronic LV failure.[42,43] However, a prospective randomized clinical trial with prostacyclin and left heart failure suggested worsening survival in the treated group for reasons that remain unclear.[44] Current practice is to gradually uptitrate the dose of the intravenous prostacyclin in patients with PH until they develop a normal cardiac index because excessive dosing of prostacyclin has been shown to cause high-output cardiac failure.[41] Often, increasing the prostacyclin dose will have little effect on the pulmonary artery pressure. Recently published studies suggest that prostacyclins do not protect the pulmonary vasculature against developing advanced disease in patients with PH, but they are able to maintain relatively normal RV function even in the face of severe pulmonary vascular disease.[25] This important observation would indicate that a new treatment paradigm that focuses on the preservation of RV function rather than the reversal of the vascular disease may be worth testing in PH. In this regard, prostacyclin may be a preferred treatment of PH in patients who present with RV failure.

SUMMARY

Clinical trials to evaluate therapies of chronic PH have largely ignored right ventricular function. Not only are there little data characterizing baseline RV function in these patients, but the selection of possible treatments have failed to address the potential beneficial or detrimental effects on RV function with treatment. As clinical studies have convincingly shown that RV function is a key determinant of long-term clinical outcome and survival in patients with PH,[45] future trials need to use biochemical, functional, and imaging modalities to characterize the RV and its response to therapy.

REFERENCES

1. Brickner ME, Hillis LD, Lange RA, et al. Congenital heart disease in adults. N Engl J Med 2000;342: 256–63.
2. Vlahakes GJ, Turley K, Hoffman JIE. The pathophysiology of failure in acute right ventricular hypertension: hemodynamic and biochemical correlations. Circulation 1981;63:87–95.
3. Klima UP, Lee M, Guerrero JL, et al. Determinants of maximal right ventricular function: role of septal shift. J Thorac Cardiovasc Surg 2002;123:72–80.
4. Saleh S, Liakopoulos OJ, Buckberg GD. The septal motor of biventricular function. Eur J Cardiothorac Surg 2006;29:S126–38.
5. Pennell DJ. Cardiovascular magnetic resonance. Circulation 2010;12:692–705.
6. Laughlin MH. Cardiovascular response to exercise. Am J Physiol 1999;277:S244–59.
7. Haddad F, Doyle R, Murphy DJ, et al. Right ventricular function in cardiovascular disease, part ii. pathophysiology, clinical importance, and management of right ventricular failure. Circulation 2008;117:1717–31.
8. Haddad F, Ashley E, Michelakis E. New insights for the diagnosis and management of right ventricular failure, from molecular imaging to targeted right ventricular therapy. Curr Opin Cardiol 2010;25: 131–40.
9. Akazawa H, Komuro I. Roles of cardiac transcription factors in cardiac hypertrophy. Circ Res 2003;92: 1079–88.
10. Hilfiker-Kleiner D, Landmesser U, Drexler H. Molecular mechanisms in heart failure. Focus on cardiac hypertrophy, inflammation, angiogenesis, and apoptosis. J Am Coll Cardiol 2006;48:A56–66.
11. Williams L, Frenneaux M. Diastolic ventricular interaction: from physiology to clinical practice. Nat Clin Pract Cardiovasc Med 2006;3:368–76.
12. Santamore WP, Burkhoff D. Hemodynamic consequences of ventricular interaction as assessed by model analysis. Am J Physiol 1991;260:H146–57.
13. Nootens M, Wolfkiel C, Chomka EV, et al. Understanding right and left ventricular systolic function and interactions at rest and with exercise in primary pulmonary hypertension. Am J Cardiol 1995;73: 379–84.
14. D'Alonzo GE, Barst RJ, Ayres SM, et al. Survival in patients with primary pulmonary hypertension. Results from a national prospective registry. Ann Intern Med 1991;115:343–9.
15. Alpert JS. The effect of right ventricular dysfunction on left ventricular form and function. Chest 2001; 119:1632–3.

16. Gan CT, Lankhaar JW, Marcus JT, et al. Impaired left ventricular filling due to right-to-left ventricular interaction in patients with pulmonary arterial hypertension. Am J Physiol Heart Circ Physiol 2006;290: H1528–33.

17. Gurudevan SV, Malouf PJ, Auger WR, et al. Abnormal left ventricular diastolic filling in chronic thromboembolic pulmonary hypertension: true diastolic dysfunction or left ventricular underfilling? J Am Coll Cardiol 2007;49:1334–9.

18. Filusch A, Giannitsis E, Katus HA, et al. High-sensitive troponin T: a novel biomarker for prognosis and disease severity in patients with pulmonary arterial hypertension. Clin Sci (Lond) 2010;119:207–13.

19. Lowensohn HS, Khouri EM, Gregg DE, et al. Phases right coronary artery blood flow in conscious dogs with normal and elevated right ventricular pressures. Circ Res 1976;39:760–6.

20. Brian C, Williams AG Jr, Gwirtz PA, et al. Right coronary autoregulation in conscious, chronically instrumented dogs. Am J Physiol Heart Circ Physiol 1998;275:H169–75.

21. Bogaard HJ, Natarajan R, Henderson SC, et al. Chronic pulmonary artery pressure elevation is insufficient to explain right heart failure. Circulation 2009;120:1951–60.

22. Gomez A, Bialostozky D, Zajarias A, et al. Right ventricular ischemia in patients with primary pulmonary hypertension. J Am Coll Cardiol 2001;38: 1137–42.

23. Michelakis ED, McMurtry MS, Wu X-C, et al. Dichloroacetate, a metabolic modulator, prevents and reverses chronic hypoxic pulmonary hypertension in rats: role of increased expression and activity of voltage-gated potassium channels. Circulation 2002;105:244–50.

24. Archer SL, Gomberg-Maitland M, Maitland M, et al. Mitochondrial metabolism, redox signaling, and fusion: a mitochondria-ROS-HIF-1alpha-Kv1.5 O2-sensing pathway at the intersection of pulmonary hypertension and cancer. Am J Physiol Heart Circ Physiol 2008;294:H570–8.

25. Rich S, Pogoriler J, Husain A, et al. Long-term effects of epoprostenol on the pulmonary vasculature in idiopathic pulmonary arterial hypertension. Chest 2010;138:1234–9.

26. Rehlman J, Archer SL. A proposed mitochondrial-metabolic mechanism for initiation and maintenance of pulmonary arterial hypertension in fawn-hooded rats: the Warburg model of pulmonary arterial hypertension. Adv Exp Med Biol 2010;661:171–85.

27. Rich S, Kaufman E, Levy PS. The effect of high doses of calcium-channel blockers on survival in primary pulmonary hypertension. N Engl J Med 1992;327:76.

28. Sitbon O, Humbert M, Jais X, et al. Long-term response to calcium channel blockers in idiopathic pulmonary arterial hypertension. Circulation 2005; 211:3105–11.

29. Yuan J, Aldinger A, Juhaszova M, et al. Dysfunctional voltage-gated K+ channels in pulmonary artery smooth muscle cells of patients with primary pulmonary hypertension. Circulation 1998;98: 1400–6.

30. Mandegar M, Yuan J. Role of K+ channels in pulmonary hypertension. Vasc Pharmacol 2002;38:25–33.

31. Rich S, McLaughlin VV. Endothelin receptor blockers in cardiovascular disease. Circulation 2003;108: 2184–90.

32. Krum H, Liew D. Current status of endothelin blockade for the treatment of cardiovascular and pulmonary vascular disease. Curr Opin Investig Drugs 2003;4:298–302.

33. Packer M, McMurray J, Massie BM, et al. Clinical effects of endothelin receptor antagonism with bosentan in patients with severe chronic heart failure: results of a pilot study. J Card Fail 2005;11:12–20.

34. Dupuis J, Hoeper MM. Endothelin receptor antagonists in pulmonary arterial hypertension. Eur Respir J 2008;31:407–15.

35. Nagendran J, Archer SL, Soliman D, et al. Phosphodiesterase type 5 is highly expressed in the hypertrophied human right ventricle, and acute inhibition of phosphodiesterase type 5 improves contractility. Circulation 2007;116:238–48.

36. Archer SL, Michelakis ED. Phosphodiesterase type 5 inhibitors for pulmonary arterial hypertension. N Engl J Med 2009;361:1864–71.

37. Michelakis ED, Tymchak W, Noga M, et al. Long-term treatment with oral sildenafil is safe and improves functional capacity and hemodynamics in patients with pulmonary arterial hypertension. Circulation 2003;108:2066–9.

38. Galie N, Ghofrani HA, Torbicki A, et al. Sildenafil citrate therapy for pulmonary arterial hypertension. N Engl J Med 2005;353:2148–57.

39. Simonneau G, Rubin LJ, Galiè N, et al. Addition of sildenafil to long-term intravenous epoprostenol therapy in patients with pulmonary arterial hypertension: a randomized trial. Ann Intern Med 2008;149: 521–30.

40. Moncada S. Prostacyclin, from discovery to clinical application. J Pharmacol 1985;16:71.

41. Rich S, McLaughlin V. The effects of chronic prostacyclin therapy on cardiac output and symptoms in primary pulmonary hypertension. J Am Coll Cardiol 1999;34:1184–7.

42. McLaughlin VV, Shillington A, Rich S. Survival in primary pulmonary hypertension: the impact of epoprostenol therapy. Circulation 2002;106:1477–82.

43. Sitbon O, Humbert M, Nunes H, et al. Long-term intravenous epoprostenol infusion in primary pulmonary hypertension: prognostic factors and survival. J Am Coll Cardiol 2002;40:780–8.

44. Califf RM, Adams KF, McKenna WJ, et al. A randomized controlled trial of epoprostenol therapy for severe congestive heart failure: the Flolan International Randomized Survival Trial (FIRST). Am Heart J 1997;134:44–54.

45. Van de Veerdonk MC, Kind T, Marcus JT, et al. Progressive right ventricular dysfunction in patients with pulmonary arterial hypertension responding to therapy. J Am Coll Cardiol 2011;58: 2511–9.

Right Ventricular Performance in Chronic Congestive Heart Failure

Gabriel T. Sayer, MD, Marc J. Semigran, MD*

KEYWORDS

- Right ventricle • Right ventricular failure
- Right ventricular dysfunction • Ventricular interdependence
- Pulmonary hypertension • Right heart catheterization
- Phosphodiesterase-5 inhibitors

Key Points

- Right ventricular anatomy and physiology are distinct from left ventricular anatomy and physiology.
- The right ventricle (RV) is able to accommodate large changes in preload but is highly afterload sensitive.
- Right ventricular hemodynamics can adversely affect left ventricular hemodynamics through ventricular interdependence.
- Right ventricular dysfunction can occur as a result of intrinsic myocardial disease, volume overload, pressure overload, or a combination of these factors.
- Right ventricular dysfunction is associated with impaired exercise capacity and worse survival.
- Multiple noninvasive modalities can be used to image the RV, with cardiac magnetic resonance imaging (MRI) being the preferred technique because of its ability to accurately measure right ventricular volumes and function.
- Right heart catheterization can differentiate the causes of right ventricular failure and aid in the management strategy.
- Treatment of right ventricular failure relies on targeting therapies toward specific causative factors as well as optimizing preload, afterload, and contractility.

The RV has historically been underrepresented in the medical literature exploring cardiac structure, function, and pathophysiology. Early research fostered the misconception that the RV played a passive role in the maintenance of cardiac output. The success of procedures to treat congenital heart disease, such as the Fontan operation, in which the RV was excluded from the venous return to the heart, also suggested that the RV contribution to normal cardiac function was limited. A lack of adequate noninvasive imaging modalities further hindered the study of RV anatomy and physiology.

As a result, understanding of the RV's contribution to cardiac disease processes has lagged behind the wealth of data about the left ventricle (LV).

In recent years, an appreciation of the central position that the RV holds in the pathophysiology of congestive heart failure has fueled interest in RV structure and function. This increased interest has coincided with the refinement of two-dimensional echocardiography, the development of three-dimensional echocardiography, and, most importantly, the growth of cardiac MRI. These imaging techniques provide a more comprehensive

---

Cardiology Division, Department of Medicine, Massachusetts General Hospital and Harvard Medical School, 55 Fruit Street, GRB-800, Boston, MA 02114, USA
* Corresponding author.
E-mail address: msemigran@partners.org

Cardiol Clin 30 (2012) 271–282
doi:10.1016/j.ccl.2012.03.011
0733-8651/12/$ – see front matter © 2012 Elsevier Inc. All rights reserved.

picture of the RV than was previously possible, and have facilitated the collection of both cross-sectional and longitudinal data about RV performance in patients with congestive heart failure (CHF). Multiple studies have now shown the strong association of RV function with both mortality and morbidity in chronic CHF. As a consequence of the increased focus on the RV, there has been renewed interest in developing therapies to target RV performance, primarily through interventions in the pulmonary circulation.

RIGHT VENTRICULAR STRUCTURE AND PHYSIOLOGY
Anatomy

The RV is a thin-walled structure located anterior to the LV in the chest. It is composed of 3 anatomic divisions[1]:

- Inlet from the right atrium
- RV apex
- Infundibulum, also called the outflow tract.

Unlike the LV, which is cylindrical in cross section, the RV has a crescentic shape, which complicates geometric assumptions for the calculation of ventricular volumes. Further distinguishing features of the RV include[2]:

- Prominent trabeculations
- Moderator band
- Apical displacement of the tricuspid valve
- A muscular fold separating the 2 valves.

The ventricular septum is shared, and there are muscular fibers in continuity between the LV and RV, linking the physiology of the 2 ventricles together.[3] In normal loading conditions, the septum is displaced into the RV throughout the cardiac cycle.

Physiology

RV contraction begins in the inlet and proceeds sequentially through the ventricle, terminating in the infundibulum.[4] Unlike the LV, which contracts circumferentially, the primary result of RV contraction is shortening of the longitudinal axis. In addition, active contraction of the RV free wall draws it inward toward the septum. LV contraction also contributes to RV contractility through force transmitted by the shared septal fibers. Because the RV has a larger end-diastolic volume than the LV, the RV ejection fraction (RVEF) is typically lower than the LV ejection fraction (LVEF).

The pressure-volume relationship of the RV differs from that of the LV (**Fig. 1**). Most notably, RV pressure begins to decline before closure of the pulmonic valve, leading to a trapezoidal configuration of the RV pressure-volume loop.[5,6] The RV continues to eject blood despite a decline in pressure because it is coupled with the high compliance and low resistance of the pulmonary vasculature. As a result, the RV is able to produce the same cardiac output as the LV with markedly less myocardial work.[2] However, one consequence of this aspect of RV physiology is a heightened sensitivity to increases in afterload. With increases in the pulmonary vascular resistance (PVR), the pressure-volume loop takes on a rectangular configuration that is similar to the pressure-volume loop of the LV.[7]

Another distinguishing feature of the RV is its ability to accommodate varying degrees of preload while maintaining a stable cardiac output.[8] Two characteristics of the RV structure permit this adaptation: the distensibility of its free wall

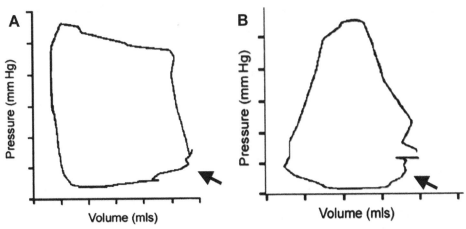

Fig. 1. Examples of simultaneous pressure and volume measurements for the LV (*A*) and RV (*B*) during a cardiac cycle. Arrowheads indicate end-diastole. (*Adapted from* Redington AN. Right ventricular function. Cardiol Clin 2002;20:342; with permission.)

and the ability to increase volume without significant changes in the wall surface area.[9] The RV does rely on the Frank-Starling mechanism to augment cardiac output, but this only occurs after a large increase in volume. In comparison, the LV has a much steeper pressure response to changes in volume. Dilation of the RV caused by volume overload is well tolerated. However, one result of chronic distention of the RV is dilation of the tricuspid valve annulus, which leads to tricuspid regurgitation. This dilation may perpetuate or worsen the chronic volume overload state. However, a reduction in cardiac output typically does not occur until the ability to tolerate further increases in preload is limited by ventricular interdependence.

Ventricular Interdependence

Early physiologic studies in a canine model erroneously suggested that the RV contribution to cardiac output was minimal.[10,11] These studies were performed without an intact pericardium, and failed to fully account for the dynamic interaction between the 2 ventricles. Because of the common pericardial sac, as well as the shared septal muscular fibers, the size and contractile state of one ventricle directly influences the function of the other ventricle. This effect is most commonly described in the context of severe RV volume overload states, which result in a shift of the ventricular septum into the LV, and consequent reduction of LV diastolic volume and cardiac output (**Fig. 2**). Systolic interactions between the 2 ventricles are intertwined as well, because the shared septal muscle fibers permit the LV to contribute energy to RV contraction.[12]

PATHOPHYSIOLOGY OF RIGHT VENTRICULAR FAILURE
Causes of Right Ventricular Dysfunction

RV dysfunction and failure is a consequence of 3 general pathophysiologic mechanisms:

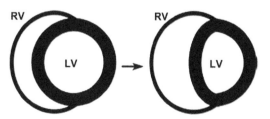

Fig. 2. Anatomic relationship of the RV and LV. The diagram on the left represents this relationship during normal loading conditions. The diagram on the right illustrates septal flattening in the context of RV volume overload. (*Reprinted from* Greyson CR. Pathophysiology of right ventricular failure. Crit Care Med 2008;36(Suppl 1):S58; with permission.)

- Intrinsic myocardial disease
- Volume overload
- Pressure overload.

Conditions leading to each of these mechanisms are listed in **Box 1**. The most common cause of RV dysfunction and failure is LV dysfunction and failure. In this context, RV dysfunction may be related to the underlying myopathy that has caused the LV to fail, as well as to the pressure load caused by increased left-sided

---

Box 1
Causes of chronic RV dysfunction and failure

Intrinsic myocardial disease
Cardiomyopathy
   Idiopathic
   Viral
   Familial
   Ischemic
   Infiltrative
Arrhythmogenic RV dysplasia

Volume overload
Tricuspid valve regurgitation
   Infective endocarditis
   Rheumatic
   Carcinoid
   Traumatic
Pulmonic valve regurgitation
Congenital heart disease
   Atrial septal defect
   Ebstein anomaly
   Anomalous pulmonary venous return

Pressure overload
Pulmonary venous hypertension
   Left heart failure
   Pulmonary venoocclusive disease
Pulmonary arterial hypertension
Hypoxia-associated PH
Chronic thromboembolic PH
Congenital heart disease
   Tetralogy of Fallot
   Pulmonic stenosis
   L-transposition of the great arteries
   Pulmonary artery stenosis
   Eisenmenger syndrome

filling pressures and consequent venous pulmonary hypertension (PH). A second common cause of RV failure is congenital heart disease, resulting in either chronic volume overload (as with an atrial septal defect) or chronic pressure overload (as with pulmonic stenosis). A detailed discussion of the pathophysiology of individual congenital heart lesions is beyond the scope of this review.

Intrinsic RV Myocardial Disease

Intrinsic myocardial disease is not typically limited to the RV. With most non-ischemic cardiomyopathies there is biventricular involvement, making it difficult to separate how much of the right-sided failure is related to left-sided failure and how much is caused by intrinsic RV dysfunction. Isolated RV dysfunction can be seen with arrhythmogenic right ventricular dysplasia but this disease usually manifests through ventricular arrhythmias rather than RV failure. In animal models, reduced RV contractility in the setting of a normal PVR does not cause a decline in cardiac output.[13] In this situation, flow through the pulmonary circuit is maintained by higher central filling pressures. However, in the context of an increased PVR, RV failure quickly ensues. Thus, intrinsic myocardial processes contribute to RV dysfunction, but an additional stressor may be necessary to provoke RV failure.

Response of the RV to Volume Overload

Chronic excess volume is well tolerated by the RV because of its ability to adapt to changes in preload without a significant increase in pressure. One consequence of RV dilatation is distortion of the architecture of the tricuspid valve and worsening tricuspid regurgitation, which may worsen the volume overload. In time, pulmonary pressures increase because of excess flow, and may be the tipping point that pushes patients with volume overload states into decompensation.[14] In an animal model, animals with volume overload alone had normal contractility, but were unable to augment their contractility appropriately when faced with the additional burden of an increased afterload.[15] As discussed earlier, one ultimate consequence of prolonged volume overload is a reduction in cardiac output caused by septal shifting and impairment of LV performance.

Response of the RV to Pressure Overload

Because of the sensitivity of the RV to increases in afterload, small increases in pulmonary arterial pressure have greater effects on RV performance than those of the LV (**Fig. 3**).[16] As with a massive

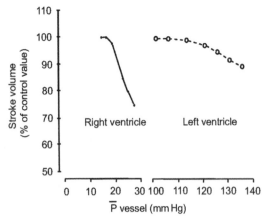

Fig. 3. Response of canine right ventricular and left ventricular stroke volume to acute changes in afterload. (*Reprinted from* Abel FL, Waldhausen JA. Effects of alterations in pulmonary vascular resistance on right ventricular function. J Thorac Cardiovasc Surg 1967;54:886; with permission.)

pulmonary embolism, acute RV pressure overload leads to rapid RV failure and may result in hemodynamic collapse. However, when pressure overload develops gradually, a series of adaptations permit short-term compensation:

- Myocyte hypertrophy allows the generation of sufficient force to deliver blood into the pulmonary circuit
- RV dilation and transformation into a more spherical configuration reduces wall stress
- Rising central venous pressure maintains cardiac output via the Frank-Starling mechanism.

The compensatory mechanisms lead to a mismatch between myocardial blood supply and oxygen demand, which increases due to wall stress when the ventricle dilates. The development of RV hypertrophy ameliorates wall stress, but, because coronary blood flow is unable to match the increased demand of hypertrophied myocardium, myocardial contractile reserve is overwhelmed and RV failure ensues (**Fig. 4**).[17] One clinical indication of advanced RV failure is a reduction in the pulmonary artery (PA) pressure coincident with a decrease in cardiac index caused by insufficient power generation by the RV.

Changes that occur at the cellular level in pressure overload states include:

- Proliferation of cardiomyoctyes[18,19]
- Increase in myocardial connective tissue[18,19]
- Downregulation of α-myosin heavy chain production and reversion to a fetal gene pattern with dominance of β-myosin heavy chain[19,20]

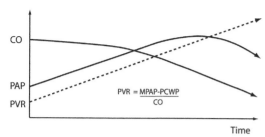

Fig. 4. Changes in hemodynamics over time with a progressive increase in RV afterload. CO, cardiac output; MPAP, mean pulmonary artery pressure; PAP, pulmonary artery pressure; PCWP, pulmonary artery capillary wedge pressure. (*Reprinted from* Haddad F, Doyle R, Murphy DJ, et al. Right ventricular function in cardiovascular disease, Part II. Circulation 2008;117: 1721; with permission.)

- Increased collagen synthesis and the development of fibrosis[21]
- Upregulation of the sympathetic nervous, endothelin and renin-angiotensin-aldosterone systems.[18,22,23]

CLINICAL SIGNIFICANCE OF RIGHT VENTRICULAR FAILURE
RV Function and Morbidity

RV dysfunction plays a crucial role in the functional capacity of patients with heart failure. Exercise capacity, as measured by peak oxygen consumption, strongly predicts mortality in heart failure.[24] Although LVEF correlates poorly with exercise capacity, RVEF is a potent predictor of both peak oxygen consumption and percent of maximum oxygen consumption achieved during cardiopulmonary exercise testing.[25,26] Furthermore, poor RV performance has also been associated with the presence of ventilatory inefficiency (slope of ventilation [VE]/CO_2 output [V_{CO_2}]) during exercise.[27] However, the relationship between RV function and exercise capacity has not been consistent across all studies, perhaps because of the heterogeneous nature of the patients who have been studied, and small sample sizes.[28,29]

The consequences of RV failure can extend to other organ systems. Prolonged increase of the central venous pressure caused by right ventricular failure may lead to hepatic congestion and dysfunction, and ultimately result in cirrhosis. Increased right-sided filling pressures have also been implicated in the cardiorenal syndrome and may be the dominant mechanism of impaired renal function in chronic heart failure.[30,31] Intestinal edema can impair absorption of nutrients, leading to malnutrition. It may also affect the bioavailability of oral medications, decreasing their therapeutic effect. In addition, chronic lower extremity edema may lead to venous insufficiency and venous ulcerations.

RV Function and Mortality

Multiple investigations have shown a strong correlation between RV function and heart failure mortality.[25,32–37] This finding has been consistent in both ischemic and nonischemic cardiomyopathies.[32,33] In 3 of these studies, RVEF had a stronger prognostic value than LVEF.[25,33,35] The degree of PH, in the presence of either a normal LVEF or a reduced LVEF, also correlates with mortality, presumably because of the effect of PH on RV function.[38] In a study of patients with chronic heart failure, patients who had both RV dysfunction and PH had worse outcomes than patients with either of these findings in isolation, suggesting that RV dysfunction and PH have an additive effect in their contribution to mortality (**Fig. 5**).[35]

EVALUATION OF RIGHT VENTRICULAR FUNCTION AND RIGHT VENTRICULAR FAILURE

A thorough history and comprehensive physical examination are integral to the assessment of RV failure. Attention should be directed to evidence of right-sided volume overload, including ascites and peripheral edema, as well as the identification of factors that may have precipitated decompensation. Further information can be provided by both noninvasive and invasive techniques. RV performance is more challenging to characterize noninvasively than LV performance. Many of the imaging methods used to assess the RV are load dependent, and may not accurately reflect the underlying RV function. Modalities that can precisely calculate RV volumes, particularly cardiac MRI, provide the most comprehensive information, and have become the gold standard in the noninvasive evaluation of the RV. However, hemodynamic assessment with cardiac catheterization is often necessary to fully characterize the cause and status of RV dysfunction. **Table 1** summarizes the advantages and disadvantages of the modalities that are commonly used to measure RV performance.

Radionuclide Ventriculography

Radionuclide ventriculography can be performed using either first-pass or equilibrium techniques. First-pass ventriculography permits the separation of the RV from the right atrium, allowing an accurate assessment of RV volume throughout the cardiac cycle.[39] Radionuclide imaging is count

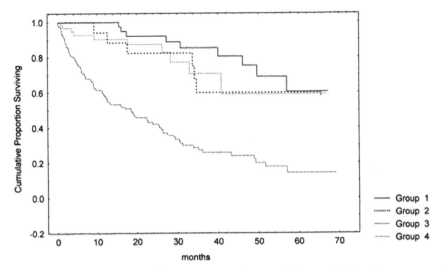

Fig. 5. Survival curves for patients grouped by presence or absence of abnormal PAP and presence or absence of abnormal RVEF. Group 1 patients had a normal PAP and RVEF. Group 2 patients had a normal PAP with a low RVEF. Group 3 patients had an increased PAP with a normal RVEF. Group 4 patients had an increased PAP and a low RVEF. Survival was significantly worse for patients with abnormalities of both PAP and RVEF. (*Reprinted from* Ghio S, Gavazzi A, Campana C et al. Independent and additive prognostic value of right ventricular systolic function and PA pressure in patients with chronic heart failure. J Am Coll Cardiol 2001;37:187; with permission.)

based, obviating geometric assumptions. Although it provides an accurate assessment of RV volumes and RVEF, its use is limited by the lack of additional information provided, including valvular abnormalities, hemodynamics, and PA pressures. In addition, availability of the equipment to perform first-pass radionuclide ventriculography, including a multicrystal γ camera and appropriate software, is limited.

Echocardiography

Two-dimensional echocardiography is the most readily accessible imaging technique for evaluating RV function and physiology. Using multiple views, including M-mode, dimensions of the inflow and outflow of the main body can be obtained, although the complex anatomy of the RV precludes accurate calculation of volumes from these measurements.[40,41] Often, the size of the RV is judged qualitatively, with the LV being used as a standard for comparison. Three-dimensional echocardiography offers the ability to calculate RV volumes and RVEF, although studies have reported a varying degree of correlation with MRI.[42,43] Echocardiography is particularly useful for measuring the degree of tricuspid regurgitation and estimating the PA pressure. Imaging of the inferior vena cava and hepatic veins can provide additional information about the diastolic pressure in the right atrium and RV.

The echocardiographic assessment of RV function is complicated by the geometry of the RV and by the sensitivity of the RVEF to changes in loading conditions. Several quantitative methods have been developed to aid in the functional assessment of the RV. The RV fractional area change is calculated as the ratio of systolic area change to diastolic area, as measured in the apical 4-chamber view. This measure correlates well with MRI-assessed RVEF, and is inversely associated with adverse outcomes in patients with LV dysfunction following a myocardial infarction.[44–46] The tricuspid annular peak systolic excursion (TAPSE), measures the vertical motion of the tricuspid annulus, reflecting that RV contraction primarily occurs in the longitudinal axis. A reduced TAPSE is associated with mortality in PH, acute myocardial infarction, and chronic heart failure.[47–49]

Two Doppler echocardiographic techniques that do not rely on geometric assumptions are isovolumic myocardial acceleration (IVA) and the RV myocardial performance index (Tei index).[50,51] IVA is the maximal isovolumic myocardial velocity divided by the time to peak velocity. The Tei index is the sum of isovolumic contraction and relaxation time divided by the time for ventricular ejection. These indices provide a measurement of RV function that is independent of loading conditions, and may therefore be a more accurate estimate of underlying RV contractility.[1,52] In both isolated PH and chronic heart failure, the Tei index has been associated with adverse outcomes.[53,54]

Table 1
Advantages and disadvantages of selected noninvasive imaging modalities for the assessment of RV function

Type of Imaging Modality	Advantages	Disadvantages
Radionuclide ventriculography	Accurate calculation of RVEF Does not require geometric assumptions	Limited availability of equipment Poor spatial resolution No information on valve function Cannot measure pulmonary pressures
Two-dimensional echocardiography	Good spatial and temporal resolution Readily available Portable and easy to use Inexpensive Safe Excellent assessment of valve function	Requires geometric assumptions for calculation of RVEF Dependent on adequate acoustic window Calculation of RVEF is highly load dependent Limited information about pulmonary arterial system
Three-dimensional echocardiography	Can measure full RV volumes without geometric assumptions	Limited temporal resolution Subject to artifact with arrhythmias because of averaging of multiple cardiac cycles Additional image processing required
Magnetic resonance imaging	Good spatial and temporal resolution Can obtain images in multiple orientations Reproducible Gold standard for calculation of RV volumes and RVEF Provides information about valvular flow, pulmonary flow, shunt fractions, and cardiac output	Not widely available Cost Requires high level of technical expertise for performance and interpretation Not compatible with pacemakers or ICDs Contraindicated in patients with renal failure

Abbreviations: ICD, implantable cardiac defibrillator; NSF, nephrogenic systemic fibrosis.

MRI

MRI has become the preferred imaging test for evaluation of the RV because of its excellent spatial and temporal resolution, as well as its ability to accurately measure volumes and RVEF without relying on geometric assumptions. MRI-calculated RV volumes have been associated with prognosis in chronic heart failure, idiopathic pulmonary arterial hypertension, and congenital heart disease.[55–57] MRI provides a wealth of diagnostic information, including quantification of hypertrophy, the evaluation of infiltrative processes (such as fibrofatty infiltration in arrhythmogenic right ventricular dysplasia), and the identification of patterns of fibrosis through delayed contrast enhancement. Furthermore, MRI offers hemodynamic evaluation of the RV and pulmonary circulation, as well as the interaction between the RV and LV. Use of MRI is limited by its cost and the requirement for technical expertise. A major limitation often encountered in the evaluation of heart failure patients\is the incompatibility of the magnetic field with common medical devices, such as pacemakers and implantable cardiac defibrillators. The development of devices resistant to a magnetic field[58] may permit more extensive use of MRI for cardiac imaging of patients with heart failure in the future.

Cardiac Catheterization

Direct measurement of intracardiac pressures during right heart catheterization remains the most accurate method of determining RV preload, afterload, and contractility. Catheterization can provide both diagnostic and therapeutic information, as well as longitudinal tracking of response to therapy. In particular, measurement of the right atrial (RA) pressure, PA pressure and pulmonary capillary wedge pressure (PCWP) may clarify the cause of RV failure (**Table 2**). Cases of isolated RV failure, as seen with diseases of the pulmonic or tricuspid valve, have an increased RA pressure with normal PA pressure and PCWP. Cardiac output may be normal or reduced.

When the PA pressure is increased, the PCWP can help to differentiate precapillary PH from postcapillary PH. Low PCWP in the setting of high pulmonary pressures is usually diagnostic of pulmonary arterial hypertension (PAH). An increased PCWP (≥15 mm Hg) suggests that the PH is caused by left-sided heart failure, mediated through pulmonary venous congestion. The transpulmonary gradient (TPG) can provide further diagnostic information.[59] When the TPG is low (<10–12 mm Hg), the PH is termed passive, indicating a pure postcapillary contribution to the elevated pulmonary pressures. When TPG is increased (usually >15 mm Hg), this indicates the presence of precapillary PH, a result of both pulmonary arterial remodeling following prolonged exposure to increased pressures and active vasoconstriction in response to increased pulmonary venous pressure. This situation is categorized as mixed PH and is further divided into patients who have reactive PH and those who have nonreactive PH. In reactive PH, acute administration of a pulmonary vasodilator, such as sodium nitroprusside, nitroglycerin, inhaled nitric oxide, or milrinone, reduces the TPG in addition to reducing left-sided pressures. In nonreactive PH, the TPG remains increased despite a reduction in the PCWP. The presence of reactivity to an acute vasodilator has been used to identify heart failure patients with PH and LV systolic dysfunction who will not suffer from RV failure after cardiac transplantation.[60] It may suggest the possibility that the patient will benefit from chronic pulmonary

vasodilator therapy, although this hypothesis remains to be proved.

Calculation of the PVR provides the best clinical estimate of RV afterload, and can be used to monitor chronic response to therapy. More sophisticated assessment of RV afterload can be determined from time-domain and frequency-domain analysis of pulmonary arterial pressure; however, this is currently only available in the research setting.[61] Frequency-domain analysis allows an inclusion in afterload measurement of the pressure wave reflected back into the main PA during late systole, which can be a significant contributor to RV afterload.

MANAGEMENT OF CHRONIC RIGHT VENTRICULAR FAILURE

Fig. 6 summarizes a general approach to the management of RV failure, which should be targeted toward the specific causative factor, as well as optimization of preload, afterload, and contractility.

Preload

Optimizing RV performance requires adequate preload to generate a sufficient stroke volume without causing a degree of RV distention that impairs LV performance through ventricular interdependence. The ideal preload required may differ between patients and will rely on both the degree of RV contractility and the severity of RV afterload. Typically, loop diuretics are the primary agents used when excessive volume is present, with the addition of thiazide diuretics as needed. In extreme circumstances, ultrafiltration or hemodialysis may be required to reduce central venous pressures. As with LV dysfunction, patients should restrict sodium and fluid intake to minimize volume retention.

Table 2
Hemodynamic profiles of different causes of RV failure

Cause of RV Failure	RAP	PAP	PCWP	TPG	PVR	Clinical Examples
Isolated RV dysfunction	↑	↓	↓	↓	↓	ARVD Pulmonic stenosis
Precapillary PH	↑	↑	↓	↓	↓	Idiopathic PAH CTEPH Hypoxia-associated PH Congenital heart disease
Passive PH (postcapillary PH)	↑	↑	↑	↓	↓	Left heart failure
Mixed PH (precapillary and postcapillary PH)	↑	↑	↑	↑	↑	Left heart failure

Abbreviations: ARVD, arrhythmogenic right ventricular dysplasia; CTEPH, chronic thromboembolic PH; PAH, pulmonary arterial hypertension; PAP, pulmonary artery pressure; RAP, right atrial pressure; TPG, transpulmonary gradient.

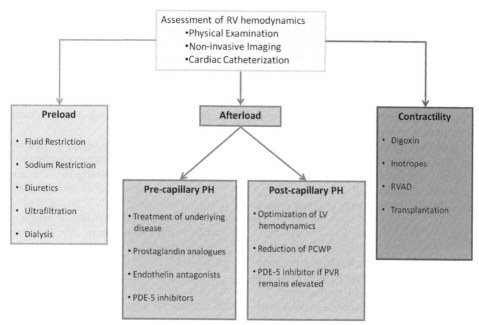

Fig. 6. Algorithm for the management of RV failure. Following diagnosis of the primary cause of RV failure, treatment should focus on optimization of preload, afterload, and contractility, as shown. ARVD, arrhythmogenic right ventricular dysplasia; CTEPH, chronic thromboembolic PH; PDE-5, phosphodiesterase-5; RAP, right atrial pressure; RVAD, right ventricular assist device.

Afterload

Reducing PA pressure is a critical component of enhancing RV performance. In all patients, persistently low oxygen saturations should be treated with supplemental oxygen to alleviate hypoxia-induced vasoconstriction. For patients with PAH, direct pulmonary vasodilators have salutary hemodynamic benefits, primarily a reduction in PA pressures, as well as significant reductions in disease-related morbidity, presumably caused by augmentation of RV function.[62,63] Three classes of pharmacologic agents are approved for the treatment of PAH: prostaglandins, endothelin antagonists, and phosphodiesterase-5 inhibitors (PDE-5Is).

For PH that is secondary to left ventricular dysfunction, initial therapy should be directed at optimizing left-sided filling pressures and thus reducing the passive component of the PH. If the PVR remains increased despite the lowering of left-sided pressures, consideration can be given to therapies that preferentially target the pulmonary vasculature. Sildenafil, a PDE-5I, has been shown to reduce PVR without significant changes in the systemic blood pressure in patients with LV dysfunction.[64] When administered chronically, sildenafil improves exercise capacity and ventilatory efficiency in this population.[65,66] Hemodynamic benefits of sildenafil have also been shown in patients with heart failure and a preserved ejection fraction.[67] There are no outcomes data for sildenafil in patients with left-sided heart failure. The benefits of sildenafil in postcapillary PH do not extend to the other agents used in the management of PAH (prostaglandins and endothelin antagonists), which have consistently been associated with adverse effects in patients with LV failure.[68–70] Novel agents, such as riociguat, a soluble guanylate cyclase stimulator, are currently being investigated for the treatment of RV dysfunction in heart failure (NCT 01065454).

Contractility

Despite optimization of loading conditions, RV failure may persist because of severe contractile dysfunction. In these situations, inotropic agents may provide some clinical benefit. Digoxin has shown short-term hemodynamic benefit in patients with PAH and has been used as a procontractile agent in the chronic management of RV failure, although outcomes data are lacking.[71] Dobutamine, milrinone, or dopamine can also be used to enhance cardiac output, with milrinone providing the additional benefit of pulmonary vasodilation. Chronic use of these agents has been associated with worse outcomes in patients with left-sided heart failure. In addition to its vasodilatory properties, sildenafil may also exert a positive inotropic effect on RV myocardium.[72]

When biventricular failure is refractory, mechanical circulatory support may be considered as part of a bridge-to-transplant strategy. A right ventricular assist device (RVAD) may occasionally be placed in conjunction with a left ventricular assist device (LVAD) to manage RV failure in the postoperative period. The only devices that are approved for RV support are extracorporeal, and are not meant to be used for long-term support. These devices are typically explanted once hemodynamics have improved, leaving the patient with LVAD support alone. Cardiac transplantation is the definitive treatment of patients with advanced RV failure, although this option is limited by the supply of donor organs.

SUMMARY

Despite significant progress in the overall management of CHF, most research in this area has focused on LV function and remodeling. The management of RV dysfunction remains a challenge. Recent studies have provided a clearer picture of RV physiology, enabling a better understanding of the chain of events that leads to RV failure. Furthermore, the multiple clinical studies highlighting the close correlation between RV function and outcomes have spurred an interest in developing therapies to specifically target the RV. At the same time, improvements in the quality of noninvasive imaging technologies are facilitating the measurement of relevant outcomes as well as enhancing the clinical management of patients with RV failure. Future research into both pharmacologic and mechanical therapies should provide an expanded array of therapeutic options for the enhancement of RV performance.

REFERENCES

1. Haddad F, Hunt SA, Rosenthal DN, et al. Right ventricular function in cardiovascular disease, part I. Circulation 2008;117:1436–48.
2. Sheehan F, Redington A. The right ventricle: anatomy, physiology and clinical imaging. Heart 2008;94:1510–5.
3. Dell'Italia LJ. The right ventricle: anatomy, physiology and clinical importance. Curr Probl Cardiol 1991;16:653–720.
4. Meier GD, Bove AA, Santamore WP, et al. Contractile function in canine right ventricle. Am J Physiol 1980;239:H794–804.
5. Shaver JA, Nadolny RA, O'Toole JD, et al. Sound pressure correlates of the second heart sound. An intracardiac sound study. Circulation 1974;49:316–25.
6. Redington AN, Gray HH, Hodson ME, et al. Characterisation of the normal right ventricular pressure-volume relation by biplane angiography and simultaneous micromanometer pressure measurements. Br Heart J 1988;59:23–30.
7. Borlaug BA, Kass DA. Invasive hemodynamic assessment in heart failure. Heart Fail Clin 2009;5:217–28.
8. Guazzi M, Pepi M, Maltagliati A. How the two sides of the heart adapt to a graded impedance to venous return with head-up tilting. J Am Coll Cardiol 1995;26(7):1732–40.
9. Greyson CR. Pathophysiology of right ventricular failure. Crit Care Med 2008;36(Suppl):S57–65.
10. Starr I, Jeffers WA, Meade RH. The absence of conspicuous increments of venous pressure after severe damage to the RV of the dog, with discussion of the relation between clinical congestive heart failure and heart disease. Am Heart J 1943;26:291–301.
11. Kagan A. Dynamic responses of the right ventricle following extensive damage by cauterization. Circulation 1952;5:816–23.
12. Damiano RJ Jr, La Follette P Jr, Cox JL, et al. Significant left ventricular contribution to right ventricular systolic function. Am J Physiol 1991;261:H1514–24.
13. Brooks H, Kirk ES, Vokonas PS, et al. Performance of the right ventricle under stress: relation to right coronary flow. J Clin Invest 1971;50:2176–83.
14. Webb G, Gatzoulis MA. Atrial septal defects in the adult. Circulation 2006;114:1645–53.
15. Szabo G, Soos P, Bahrle S, et al. Adaptation of the right ventricle to an increased afterload in the chronically volume overloaded heart. Ann Thorac Surg 2006;82:989–95.
16. Abel FL, Waldhausen JA. Effects of alterations in pulmonary vascular resistance on right ventricular function. J Thorac Cardiovasc Surg 1967;54:886–94.
17. Guyton AC, Lindsey AW, Gilluly JJ. The limits of right ventricular compensation following acute increase in pulmonary circulatory resistance. Circ Res 1954;2:326–32.
18. Haddad F, Doyle R, Murphy DJ, et al. Right ventricular function in cardiovascular disease, Part II. Circulation 2008;117:1717–31.
19. Bogaard HJ, Abe K, Noordegraaf AV, et al. The right ventricle under pressure: cellular and molecular mechanisms of right-heart failure in pulmonary hypertension. Chest 2009;135:794–804.
20. Lowes BD, Minobe W, Abraham WT, et al. Changes in gene expression in the intact human heart: down-regulation of alpha-myosin heavy chain in hypertrophied, failing ventricular myocardium. J Clin Invest 1997;100(9):2315–24.
21. Bishop JE, Rhodes S, Laurent GJ, et al. Increased collagen synthesis and decreased collagen degradation in right ventricular hypertrophy induced by pressure overload. Cardiovasc Res 1994;28:1581–5.
22. Nootens M, Kaufmann E, Rector T, et al. Neurohormonal activation in patients with right ventricular

failure from pulmonary hypertension: relation to hemodynamic variables and endothelin levels. J Am Coll Cardiol 1995;26:1581–5.

23. Rouleau JL, Kapuku G, Pelletier S, et al. Cardioprotective effects of ramipril and losartan in right ventricular pressure overload in the rabbit: importance of kinins and influence on angiotensin II type I receptor signaling pathway. Circulation 2001;104: 939–44.

24. Mancini DM, Eisen H, Kussmaul W, et al. Value of peak exercise oxygen consumption for optimal timing of cardiac transplantation in ambulatory patients with heart failure. Circulation 1991;83:778–86.

25. Di Salvo TG, Mathier M, Semigran MJ, et al. Preserved right ventricular ejection fraction predicts exercise capacity and survival in advanced heart failure. J Am Coll Cardiol 1995;25:1143–53.

26. Baker B, Wilen M, Boyd C, et al. Relation of right ventricular ejection fraction to exercise capacity in chronic congestive heart failure. Am J Cardiol 1985;55:1037–42.

27. Lewis GD, Shah RV, Pappagianopalas PP, et al. Determinants of ventilator efficiency in heart failure: the role of right ventricular performance and pulmonary vascular tone. Circ Heart Fail 2008;1:227–33.

28. Rubis P, Podolec P, Kopec G, et al. The dynamic assessment of right-ventricular function and its relation to exercise capacity in heart failure. Eur J Heart Fail 2010;12:260–7.

29. Clark AL, Swan JW, Laney R, et al. The role of right and left ventricular function in the ventilator response to exercise in chronic heart failure. Circulation 1994;89:2062–9.

30. Mullens W, Abrahams Z, Tang WH, et al. Importance of venous congestion for worsening of renal function in advanced decompensated heart failure. J Am Coll Cardiol 2009;53(7):589–96.

31. Testani JM, Khera AV, St John Sutton MG, et al. Effect of right ventricular function and venous congestion on cardiorenal interactions during the treatment of decompensated heart failure. Am J Cardiol 2010;105(4):511–6.

32. Juilliere Y, Barbier G, Feldmann L, et al. Additional predictive value of both left and right ventricular ejection fractions on long-term survival in idiopathic dilated cardiomyopathy. Eur Heart J 1997;18:276–80.

33. Polak JF, Holman BL, Wynne J, et al. Right ventricular ejection fraction: an indicator of increased mortality in patients with congestive heart failure associated with coronary artery disease. J Am Coll Cardiol 1983;2:217–24.

34. de Groote P, Millaire A, Foucher-Hossein C, et al. Right ventricular ejection fraction is an independent predictor of survival in patients with moderate heart failure. J Am Coll Cardiol 1998;32:948–54.

35. Ghio S, Gavazzi A, Campana C, et al. Independent and additive prognostic value of right ventricular systolic function and PA pressure in patients with chronic heart failure. J Am Coll Cardiol 2001;37:183–8.

36. Gavazzi A, Berzuini C, Campana C, et al. Value of right ventricular ejection fraction in predicting short-term prognosis of patients with severe chronic heart failure. J Heart Lung Transplant 1997;16:774–85.

37. Meyer P, Filippatos GS, Ahmed MI, et al. Effects of right ventricular ejection fraction on outcomes in chronic systolic heart failure. Circulation 2010;121: 252–8.

38. Bursi F, McNallan SM, Redfield MM, et al. Pulmonary pressures and death in heart failure. J Am Coll Cardiol 2012;59:222–31.

39. Sanz J, Fernandez-Friera L, Moral S. Imaging techniques and the evaluation of the right heart and the pulmonary circulation. Rev Esp Cardiol 2010; 63(2):209–23.

40. Lang RM, Bierig M, Devereux RB, et al. Recommendations for chamber quantification: a report from the American Society of Echocardiography's Guidelines and Standards Committee and the Chamber Quantification Writing Group, developed in conjunction with the European Association of Echocardiography, a branch of the European Society of Cardiology. J Am Soc Echocardiogr 2005;18:1440–63.

41. Jenkins C, Chan J, Bricknell K, et al. Reproducibility of right ventricular volumes and ejection fraction using real-time three-dimensional echocardiography: comparison with cardiac MRI. Chest 2007; 131(6):1844–51.

42. Kjaergaard J, Petersen CL, Kjaer A, et al. Evaluation of right ventricular volume and function by 2D and 3D echocardiography compared to MRI. Eur J Echocardiogr 2006;7:430–8.

43. Van der Zwaan H, Helbing W, McGhie J, et al. Clinical value of real-time three-dimensional echocardiography for right ventricular quantification in congenital heart disease: validation with cardiac magnetic resonance imaging. J Am Soc Echocardiogr 2010;23:134–40.

44. Anavekar NS, Gerson D, Skali H, et al. Two-dimensional assessment of right ventricular function: an echocardiographic-MRI correlative study. Echocardiography 2007;24(5):452–6.

45. Anavekar NS, Skali H, Bourgoun M, et al. Usefulness of right ventricular fractional area change to predict death, heart failure, and stroke following myocardial infarction (from the VALIANT ECHO Study). Am J Cardiol 2008;101(5):607–12.

46. Zornoff LA, Skali H, Pfeffer MA, et al. Right ventricular dysfunction and risk of heart failure and mortality after myocardial infarction. J Am Coll Cardiol 2002;39(9):1450–5.

47. Forfia PR, Fisher MR, Mathai SC, et al. Tricuspid annular displacement predicts survival in pulmonary hypertension. Am J Respir Crit Care Med 2006;174: 1034–41.

48. Engstrom AE, Vis MM, Bouma BJ, et al. Right ventricular dysfunction is an independent predictor for mortality in ST-elevation myocardial infarction patients presenting with cardiogenic shock on admission. Eur J Heart Fail 2010;12(3):276–82.

49. Kjaergaard J, Akkan D, Iversen KK, et al. Right ventricular dysfunction as an independent predictor of short- and long-term mortality in patients with heart failure. Eur J Heart Fail 2007;9(6–7):610–6.

50. Vogel M, Derrick G, White PA, et al. Validation of myocardial acceleration during isovolumic contraction as a novel noninvasive index of right ventricular contractility: comparison with ventricular pressure-volume relations in an animal model. Circulation 2002;105:1693–9.

51. Tei C, Dujardin KS, Hodge DO, et al. Doppler echocardiographic index for assessment of global right ventricular function. J Am Soc Echocardiogr 1996; 9:838–47.

52. Pavlicek M, Wahl A, Rutz T, et al. Right ventricular systolic function assessment: rank of echocardiographic methods vs. cardiac magnetic resonance imaging. Eur J Echocardiogr 2011;12(11):871–80.

53. Yeo TC, Dujardin KS, Tei C. Value of a Doppler-derived index combining systolic and diastolic time intervals in predicting outcome in primary pulmonary hypertension. Am J Cardiol 1998;81:1157–61.

54. Harjai KL, Scott L, Vivekananthan K, et al. The Tei index: a new prognostic index for patients with symptomatic heart failure. J Am Soc Echocardiogr 2002;15(9):864–8.

55. Bourantas CV, Loh HP, Bragadeesh T, et al. Relationship between right ventricular volumes measured by cardiac magnetic resonance imaging and prognosis in patients with chronic heart failure. Eur J Heart Fail 2011;13(1):52–60.

56. van Wolferen SA, Marcus JT, Boonstra A, et al. Prognostic value of right ventricular mass, volume, and function in idiopathic pulmonary arterial hypertension. Eur Heart J 2007;28(10):1250–7.

57. Knauth AL, Gauvreau K, Powell AJ, et al. Ventricular size and function assessed by cardiac MRI predict major adverse clinical outcomes late after tetralogy of Fallot repair. Heart 2008;94(2):211–6.

58. Wilkoff BL, Bello D, Taborsky M, et al. Magnetic resonance imaging in patients with a pacemaker system designed for the magnetic resonance environment. Heart Rhythm 2011;8:65–73.

59. Chatterjee NA, Lewis GD. What is the prognostic significance of pulmonary hypertension in heart failure? Circ Heart Fail 2011;4(5):541–5.

60. Costard-Jackle A, Fowler MB. Influence of preoperative pulmonary artery pressure on mortality after heart transplantation: testing of potential reversibility of pulmonary hypertension with nitroprusside is useful in defining a high risk group. J Am Coll Cardiol 1992;19:48–54.

61. Champion HC, Michelakis EF, Hassoun PM. Comprehensive invasive and noninvasive approach to the right ventricle – Pulmonary Circulation Unit. Circulation 2009;120:992–1007.

62. Barst RJ, Gibbs JS, Ghofrani HA, et al. Updated evidence-based treatment algorithm in pulmonary arterial hypertension. J Am Coll Cardiol 2009; 54(Suppl 1):S78–84.

63. Humbert M, Sitbon O, Simonneau G. Treatment of pulmonary arterial hypertension. N Engl J Med 2004;351(14):1425–36.

64. Lewis GD, Lachmann J, Camuso J, et al. Sildenafil improves exercise hemodynamics and oxygen uptake in patients with systolic heart failure. Circulation 2007;115(1):59–66.

65. Guazzi M, Samaja M, Arena R, et al. Long-term use of sildenafil in the therapeutic management of heart failure. J Am Coll Cardiol 2007;50:2136–44.

66. Lewis GD, Shah R, Shahzad K. Sildenafil improves exercise capacity and quality of life in patients with systolic heart failure and secondary pulmonary hypertension. Circulation 2007;116(14):1555–62.

67. Guazzi M, Vicenzi M, Arena R, et al. Pulmonary hypertension in heart failure with preserved ejection fraction: a target of phosphodiesterase-5 inhibition in a 1-year study. Circulation 2011;124(2):164–74.

68. Califf RM, Adams KF, McKenna WJ, et al. A randomized controlled trial of epoprostenol therapy for severe congestive heart failure: The Flolan International Randomized Survival Trial (FIRST). Am Heart J 1997;134(1):44–54.

69. Kalta PR, Moon JC, Coats AJ. Do the results of the ENABLE (Endothelin Antagonist Bosentan for Lowering Cardiac Events in Heart Failure) study spell the end for non-selective endothelin antagonism in heart failure? Int J Cardiol 2002;85(2–3):195–7.

70. Kaluski E, Cotter G, Leitman M, et al. Clinical and hemodynamic effects of bosentan dose optimization in symptomatic heart failure patients with severe systolic dysfunction, associated with secondary pulmonary hypertension – a multi-center randomized study. Cardiology 2008;109:273–80.

71. Rich S, Seidlitz M, Dodin E, et al. The short-term effects of digoxin in patients with right ventricular dysfunction from pulmonary hypertension. Chest 1998;114(3):787–92.

72. Nagendran J, Archer SL, Soliman D, et al. Phosphodiesterase type 5 is highly expressed in the hypertrophied human right ventricle, and acute inhibition of phosphodiesterase type 5 improves contractility. Circulation 2007;116:238–48.

Right Ventricular Failure After Cardiac Surgery

Gus J. Vlahakes, MD

KEYWORDS

- Right ventricle • Right ventricular failure
- Interventricular failure • Nitric oxide • Prostacyclin
- Cardiac transplantation • Cardiac assist device

Right ventricular (RV) failure remains a significant problem after cardiac surgery. It is a particular issue in patients in certain cardiac surgical settings: congenital heart disease, mitral valve disease with pulmonary hypertension, after cardiac transplantation, institution of left ventricular (LV) support, and coronary artery disease. If not considered in the surgical management plan, RV failure can be a source of major morbidity and mortality in these patients. Particularly in an era of increasing patient complexity, this remains a significant and incompletely solved clinical problem.

Very early in the study of cardiac physiology, the RV was thought to be a superfluous organ for the normal functioning of the heart. In single-ventricle congenital heart disease, the circulation functions well without active pumping in the pulmonary circulation and with the patient's circulation reconstituted with a passive pulmonary circulation. In early experiments, physiology investigators inactivated the RV by applying heat and observed little change in the overall cardiac function in experimental animal models. As learned later, in these early experiments, the thermal inactivation of the RV free wall creates a noncompliant RV against which the contractile action of the interventricular septum can continue to maintain the RV output.

In typical settings in which RV failure may be an issue, pulmonary vascular resistance is usually, but not always, elevated, and LV function may not be normal. In contrast to the LV, RV physiology has been the subject of fewer physiologic studies. However, there are studies in the early physiology literature that are of significant relevance in the contemporary management of RV failure. More than 50 years ago, Peter Salisbury[1] demonstrated in an experimental preparation that as RV systolic pressure is increased by progressive pulmonary artery constriction, RV failure eventually occurs. Although this experimental study was done over 50 years ago, the essence of the modern management of RV failure is contained in Salisbury's classic 1955 publication (**Fig. 1**). Three important experimental observations were made as part of this study. In an experimental canine preparation, the pulmonary artery was gradually and incrementally constricted until the onset of RV failure as evidenced by decreasing RV pressure and increasing central venous pressure.

1. When central aortic pressure was increased by clamping the descending aorta, RV failure was abruptly reversed.
2. The maximal RV pressure that could be generated in each experimental preparation was proportional to the systemic pressure generated.
3. By providing increased systemic pressure, considerable RV pressure work could be performed well above what the RV was able to generate under baseline conditions.

This study did not explore mechanisms beyond simple speculation, but it did stimulate later works that suggest perfusion of the RV free wall as the responsible mechanism. RV free wall ischemia occurs later during RV failure because of pressure overload, and providing additional systemic

Disclosures: None.
Harvard Medical School, Division of Cardiac Surgery, Massachusetts General Hospital, 55 Fruit Street, COX630, Boston, MA 02114-2696, USA
E-mail address: vlahakes.gus@mgh.harvard.edu

Cardiol Clin 30 (2012) 283–289
doi:10.1016/j.ccl.2012.03.010

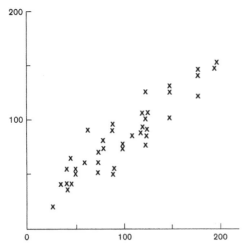

Fig. 1. Maximum systolic pressure generated by the RV during progressive pulmonary artery constriction is shown on the vertical axis. Mean femoral artery pressure is shown on the horizontal axis. (*Reproduced from Salisbury PF. Coronary artery pressure and strength of right ventricular contraction. Circ Res 1955;3:633–8; with permission.*)

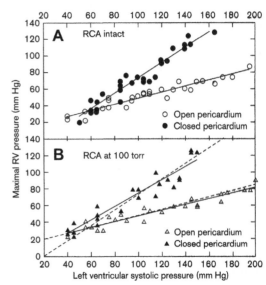

Fig. 2. The relationship between maximal developed RV pressure and LV systolic pressure under conditions of an intact right coronary artery (RCA; *A*) where right coronary perfusion pressure equals aortic pressure and under conditions of RCA perfusion pressure held constant at 100 torr (*B*). In both instances, the status of the pericardium influences the slope of the linear relations shown, that is, the status of the pericardium influences the extent to which LV systolic pressure influences maximal pressure that the RV can generate. (*Reproduced from Page RD, Harringer W, Hodakowski GT, et al. Determinants of maximal right ventricular function. J Heart Lung Transpl 1992;11:90–8; with permission.*)

perfusion pressure not only recovered RV function, but also relieved RV free wall ischemia.[2] This study suggested that maintaining RV free wall perfusion was the key clinical factor in maximizing RV function.

The analysis of the underlying physiology became more complex when it was suggested that RV performance was not simply determined by right coronary perfusion pressure. Page and colleagues[3] conducted an experimental study in a canine model. In canine experimental models, the coronary anatomy is consistently left dominant, with approximately 80% of the RV free wall perfused by a nondominant right coronary artery. In Page's study, the right coronary artery was separately cannulated and maintained at a controlled pressure. Although they demonstrated a similar relationship between systemic pressure and maximal RV pressure that could be generated, this relationship was not influenced significantly by right coronary perfusion pressure, but it was influenced by the status of the pericardium, as noted in **Fig. 2**. Page and colleagues[3] demonstrated the same linear relationship between LV systolic pressure and the maximal RV pressure that could be generated, as did other investigators. However, the slope of the linear relationship was much greater when the pericardium was left intact, strongly suggesting that some type of LV-RV interaction was an important part of RV function.

Surgical literature suggests that a significant portion of the overall RV function is derived from the interventricular septum; in an analysis of RV performance under pressure load, at least half of the RV function is derived from the interventricular septum.[4] RV preload also exerts a preloadlike function on the interventricular septum, and the developed LV pressure, not necessarily right coronary perfusion pressure, is the major determinant of the maximal potential contribution of the interventricular septum to the overall RV function.[5]

These physiologic principles have important implications for the clinical management of RV failure after cardiac surgery. Although RV failure may have different causes in different clinical settings, the management principles share similar themes:

- Minimize RV afterload.
- Optimize RV performance, including both the RV free wall and the interventricular septal contributions. This includes ensuring adequate myocardial protection during cardiac surgery.
- Hemodynamic management must therefore maximize the pressure work performed by the LV (and hence, the septal contribution to RV function) and the systemic pressure available to perfuse the RV free wall.

MONITORING PATIENTS WITH THE POTENTIAL FOR RV FAILURE

In the normal human circulation, because of the greater compliance of the RV, right atrial pressure is lower than left atrial pressure. When physiologically significant RV failure occurs, the right atrial pressure often exceeds left atrial pressure, often with a low left atrial pressure because of the inability of the right heart to provide adequate left heart filling. A minimal degree of RV failure due to a mismatched RV function and RV afterload can be defined when right atrial pressure and left atrial pressure begin to equal each other, as is frequently the case after cardiac transplantation. Although this condition might not signify overt RV failure, it suggests the need for clinical vigilance and in particular, continuous right atrial pressure and left atrial pressure monitoring, which become particularly important during the emergence from anesthesia, especially in patients who are starting out with increased pulmonary vascular resistance (PVR).

Hence, when RV failure is noted during an operation or as a potential risk, particularly after LVAD implantation or transplantation with increased PVR, a left atrial pressure line should be considered to provide continuous monitoring and continuous display of the relationship between the right-sided and left-sided filling pressures. The use of left atrial catheters in these patients provides significant information for patient management with minimal additional risk.[6]

OPERATIVE STRATEGY: CONSIDERATIONS FOR OPTIMIZING RV FUNCTION

As part of intraoperative management, consideration must be given to factors that may increase a patient's risk of RV failure and to minimize those risks. There are several strategies and patient scenarios that deserve attention.

Minimizing RV Afterload

As part of the intraoperative management of RV failure, and with particular reference to management of the pulmonary circulation, certain measures should be instituted before considering the addition of specific pulmonary vasodilators:

- The patient should be well oxygenated.
- The patient should be anesthetized and/or deeply sedated, including pharmacologic paralysis.
- Hypercarbia and acidosis should be assiduously avoided, with the goal of Pco_2 less than 40 torr.

- The pleural spaces should be free of air, blood, and effusion.
- Ventilation should be adjusted to minimize mean airway pressure:positive end expiratory pressure should be avoided and a short inspiratory time to expiratory time ratio should be used.
- The airway should be clear without mucous plugs, blood, and with a well-positioned endotracheal tube.
- Wheezing, if present, should be treated.

If these measures have been assured, and systemic hemodynamics have been optimized with a good level of developed LV pressure, pulmonary-specific vasodilation should be instituted. Most interest has been focused on this approach to manage RV failure because it is aimed at resolving what a primary pathophysiological mechanism is. Before the advent of iNO, numerous pharmacologic agents have been attempted in this setting. Although nonspecific vasodilators may reduce pulmonary vascular resistance, by reducing systemic blood pressure and hence developing LV pressure, an important determinant of maximal RV function may be adversely affected. Thus, nonspecific vasodilators, by themselves, have little role in the management of RV failure. However, one of the earliest agents used to reduce pulmonary vascular resistance in the surgical setting was prostaglandin E_1 (PGE₁).[7] Although of historical interest, this approach is still useful in settings in which contemporary agents are not available. A significant portion of the administered dose of PGE₁ administered into the systemic venous circulation is metabolized on first pass through the pulmonary circulation.[8] Thus, this can create some degree of specificity for its site of action. However, after cardiopulmonary bypass, pulmonary vascular endothelial function may be abnormal leading to greater systemic transit of vasodilator agents. Hence, when PGE₁ was used in this setting, it often required concomitant left-sided administration of norepinephrine[7] to maintain systemic pressure. This approach, although shown to be effective in this setting, is complex and requires familiarity with left atrial drug infusion. This approach was replaced by the introduction of iNO, which has provided a major improvement and simplification for the management of elevated pulmonary vascular resistance, even when potent vasoconstrictor drugs are used to maintain systemic pressure.[9]

Cost considerations have made iNO recently less popular for the management of RV failure. However, in the operating room, the ease and reliability of administration and its efficacy in this setting make iNO an ideal pharmacologic agent for the management of RV failure that prevents successful weaning from bypass. iNO is provided by the vendor as a mixture in pure nitrogen, and is introduced into the ventilator. A common starting dose is 10 ppm in the inspired gas; the dose is advanced by 5-ppm increments up to 40 ppm if needed. Although greater concentrations of iNO have been used, if there is no clinically apparent improvement at 40 ppm, additional levels of iNO will not be effective.

Once the patient is stabilized in the intensive care unit, the dose of iNO can be gradually decreased, initially, in 5-ppm increments down to 10 ppm, and thereafter in smaller increments as tolerated by pulmonary vascular resistance. If RV function is recovered, iNO can often be weaned off before extubation, or if indicated by persistent pulmonary hypertension and undesirable RV hemodynamics, use face-mask–administered iNO after extubation. One important caution is the possibility of a rebound increase in pulmonary vascular resistance after the abrupt withdrawal of iNO.[10] Thus, iNO weaning should occur with continuous monitoring of hemo-dynamics, including pulmonary artery pressure and ideally, right and left atrial pressures.

Because of concerns about the cost of iNO, other agents have entered the practice and are being used in this clinical setting. In particular, inhaled prostacyclin[11,12] has been shown to be useful in treating patients with right-sided heart failure after cardiac surgery and has been found increasingly to be an alternative agent for many patients. In patients who underwent heart and lung transplantation, it has been suggested that inhaled prostacyclin is as effective as iNO for the treatment of RV failure.[13] However, this must be administered by nebulizing it into the inspiratory gas mixture. Thus, many surgeons and critical care physicians have found it more reliable to initiate management of the pulmonary circulation with iNO, and once initial early postoperative stability has been established, to transition the patients to inhaled prostacyclin under continuous hemodynamic monitoring. Prostacyclin is nebulized into the inspiratory gas flow and can be administered via face-mask after extubation. A typical dose that is used is 30 ng/kg/min. It is usually weaned during continuous hemodynamic monitoring by decreasing the dose to 15 ng/kg/min and thereafter discontinuing its use. As with all clinical decision making, if inhaled prostacyclin is not effective in controlling pulmonary vascular resistance in patients with RV failure, management should be transitioned back to iNO.

Maximizing Function of the RV Free Wall

The previously mentioned studies on experimental physiology suggest that approximately half of overall RV function is derived from the RV free wall and half from the interventricular septum. In the setting of cardiac surgery, RV protection must be optimal, particularly for surgery in settings where RV failure is anticipated to be a risk. In concomitant coronary artery disease, the integrity of the RV blood supply must be considered. This is a typical setting in which revascularization of the RV marginal artery or arteries may be needed in the revascularization plan, not only for long-term RV perfusion but also for the short-term delivery of cardioplegia during a cardiac surgical procedure and for short-term postoperative RV perfusion.

Inotropic support should be instituted. Milrinone is a popular agent used in this setting. In addition to its inotropic effect, it can also dilate the pulmonary circulation, and it is commonly instituted before selective pulmonary vasodilation. One important issue with milrinone is its systemic vasodilator effect, and hence, its potential negative effect on the interventricular septal contribution to RV function. Thus, appropriate control of systemic vascular resistance must be incorporated into the plan selected for inotropic support of the RV free wall. Also, as noted in experimental physiologic studies, systemic perfusion pressure must be maintained to ensure RV free wall perfusion under increased pressure load, thus avoiding RV free wall ischemia.

Although the intra-aortic balloon pump (IABP) has been used to treat LV ischemia and impaired function, it has not proved to be of significant value in the treatment of RV failure. In contrast to the LV, perfusion of the right coronary artery occurs across the entire cardiac cycle; the exception is the circumstance of markedly increased pulmonary artery pressure in which the phasic pattern of RV blood flow shows diastolic predominance, as in the case of the LV. Thus, there may not be any salutary effect of IABP support on RV perfusion. Furthermore, systolic unloading of the left heart during IABP support decreases developed LV pressure, and hence may adversely affect the septal contribution to LV function.

Maximizing Left Heart Pressure Work

As shown in animal studies previously referenced, there is a significant contribution of the interventricular septum to right heart function. To this end, a strategy must be devised for each patient to wean from cardiopulmonary bypass with as much developed LV pressure as possible. In the case of a patient immediately after cardiac transplantation, this might be achieved by systemic vasoconstriction. In these patients, pretransplantation heart failure management regimens may include substantial use of vasodilator drugs for afterload reduction. In this setting, high doses of agents such as norepinephrine or vasopressin may be needed, particularly during the early postoperative hours when the effect of pretransplantation vasodilator drugs may still be present.

Patients being placed on LV assist device support

In the case of patients being placed on LV assist devices (LVAD), RV failure is a recognized complication because of the decrement in the contribution of the LV to overall RV function.[14] The risk of RV failure in this setting may be greatest in patients with poor RV function and patients with low preoperative pulmonary artery pressure, who do not experience a marked decrement in RV afterload when LV filling pressures are reduced with the institution of LVAD support.[15] Particularly in these patients, clinical management of right heart failure may be more complex. Most LVADs, when used in their automatic modes, maximally reduce LV preload and hence, LV develops pressure. In this setting, it is sometimes useful and effective to decrease LVAD flow sufficiently to allow some left heart filling and hence, increase the LV-developed pressure.

Special Considerations in Right Coronary Artery Anatomy

The nondominant right coronary artery

Patients who are undergoing cardiac surgery, particularly surgery for valvular heart disease and combined coronary artery revascularization, can present a special circumstance. The coronary circulation is not only important to ensure myocardial oxygenation for normal function but also a common route for the delivery of myocardial protection. In patients with an occluded nondominant right coronary artery, consideration must be given to ensuring the myocardial protection of the RV free wall. In this clinical circumstance, many surgeons include surgical revascularization of at least 1 RV marginal artery with the short-term goal of delivering cardioplegia and the long-term goal of providing adequate perfusion for RV function. In addition, the small right coronary ostium should still receive cardioplegia when surgery is done in the aortic valve. The addition of topical hypothermia in the form of either a cooling jacket or iced sponges may assist in enhancing RV myocardial protection. When aortic valve replacements are being done, particularly in patients with nondominant right coronary anatomy, the right coronary ostium should not be compromised. In these circumstances, particularly with a nondominant artery, RV failure is the sole manifestation of either right coronary ostium

compromise, or air embolism in the early stages of weaning cardiopulmonary bypass. A small nondominant right coronary ostium can be more vulnerable to occlusion during the seating of an aortic prosthesis. In such circumstances, the difficulty with RV function after aortic valve replacement should suggest that right coronary perfusion be assessed and bypass to the coronary artery be added if needed.

Recent right coronary artery territory infarction

Special mention is made to a particular clinical setting in which the patient has sustained an acute, right coronary territory infarction with proximal occlusion of the right coronary artery. In this circumstance, if coronary angiography does not show any patent RV marginal arteries, severe RV failure can complicate revascularization surgery. Furthermore, a patient with recent RV infarction can sometimes decompensate with anesthesia and positive pressure ventilation. This phenomenon results from the ability of the acutely infarcted RV to interfere with the filling and function of the LV, with hemodynamics that may resemble cardiac tamponade.[16] To the extent possible, such patients should be temporized by medical management and/or right coronary artery catheter intervention until RV healing and recanalization of the RV blood supply occurs. When revascularization surgery is subsequently planned, catheterization is repeated to assess the RV and should be included in preoperative evaluation, and RV marginal grafting should also be considered.

EMERGENCE FROM ANESTHESIA AND VENTILATORY WEANING

Initial emergence from anesthesia, subsequent weaning, and extubation can stress a failing RV, and RV failure may reemerge, sometimes precipitously to an extreme degree. The decision to stop sedation is should be based on the cause of right heart failure and how it has or has not improved during the initial hours of recovery after surgery.

In the setting after cardiac transplantation, decision making regarding waking up and extubation is usually straightforward. Donor heart RV function may be temporarily diminished as part of the myocardial protection and transplant process, particularly if ischemic time is long. In addition, early after transplantation, pulmonary artery pressure will not yet have reached its posttransplantation nadir. Accordingly, if right heart failure occurs after transplantation, 12 to 24 hours of additional deep sedation may be of value in stabilizing RV function and pulmonary vascular resistance and allow temporarily impaired RV function to recover.

Again, continuous monitoring of right atrial and left atrial pressures, as well as pulmonary artery pressure, is useful to detect the development of RV failure during wake up in this clinical setting.

In other clinical settings, this decision must be individualized based on the cause of RV failure and how the pathophysiology has changed during recovery. Usually, once patients are awake and extubated, spontaneous ventilation often decreases pulmonary artery pressure further, thus improving overall cardiac performance.

RV CIRCULATORY SUPPORT

When the previously discussed measures fail to stabilize the circulation to permit weaning bypass with stable hemodynamics, mechanical circulatory support should be considered. The options include RV assist device (RVAD) implantation, biventricular assist implantation, or extracorporeal membrane oxygenator (ECMO) support. The choice of mechanical support modality is determined by certain factors:

- Is RV dysfunction considered temporary?
- Is concomitant left-heart support needed?
- Is it predicted that the patient will not need support leading to transplantation?
- Is gas exchange adequate?

RVAD support is generally achieved with the same types of temporary support devices used for left-sided support. However, there is a special consideration in this setting. Contemporary ventricular assist devices are capable of delivering considerable levels of output. It is essential to ensure that the LV can tolerate significant levels of preload. Thus, concomitant measurement of left-sided filling pressure is important. It may be necessary to titrate down the level of RV support to avoid excessive LV filling pressures and pulmonary edema. Furthermore, when RVAD support is instituted, the markedly impaired RV should not be distended or it should be capable of some ejection to avoid distension and impairment of RV perfusion and recovery.

If RV function is impaired on a temporary basis from ischemia-reperfusion injury, recovery should start becoming evident at approximately 48 hours. Trials of RVAD weaning should begin when bedside hemodynamic assessment with or without echocardiography shows return of function. Often, final determination of RV recovery must be done in the operating room when RVAD support is weaned completely and preload is optimized. Once RVAD support is discontinued and the device is removed, at least an additional 24-hour period of deep sedation should be used to allow stabilization of RV function and pulmonary vascular resistance. Subsequent ventilator weaning and extubation should follow the previously described guidelines.

If concomitant left-sided support is needed, the choice of support hardware and modality depends on the adequacy of lung function. ECMO support is often useful if short-term support is needed, particularly if lung function is an issue. This can be instituted from peripheral vascular access, thus obviating reopening the chest to remove support devices.

SUMMARY

Although RV failure is an important source of morbidity and mortality after certain types of cardiac surgery, the elucidation of the details of RV physiology and the pathophysiology of RV failure have led to the development of techniques to manage this problem. Minimizing pulmonary vascular resistance, including the use of specific pulmonary vasodilators, combined with optimizing the 2 major components of RV function, the RV free wall and the interventricular septum, can stabilize many of these patients until RV function recovers and/or RV afterload decreases. In the contemporary setting, refractory RV failure can be managed by RV mechanical support.

REFERENCES

1. Salisbury PF. Coronary artery pressure and strength of right ventricular contraction. Circ Res 1955;3:633–8.
2. Vlahakes GJ, Turley K, Hoffman JI. The pathophysiology of failure in acute right ventricular hypertension; hemodynamic and biochemical correlations. Circulation 1981;63:87–95.
3. Page RD, Harringer W, Hodakowski GT, et al. Determinants of maximal right ventricular function. J Heart Lung Transplant 1992;11:90–8.
4. Klima U, Guerrero JL, Vlahakes GJ. Contribution of the interventricular septum to maximal right ventricular function. Eur J Cardiothorac Surg 1998;14:250–5.
5. Klima UP, Myung-Yong L, Guerrero JL, et al. Determinants of maximal right ventricular function: role of septal shift. J Thorac Cardiovasc Surg 2002;123:72–80.
6. Santini F, Gatti G, Borghetti V, et al. Routine left atrial catheterization for the post-operative management of cardiac surgical patients: is the risk justified? Eur J Cardiothorac Surg 1999;16:218–21.
7. D'Ambra MN, LaRaia PJ, Philbin DM, et al. Prostaglandin E_1: a new therapy for refractory right heart failure and pulmonary hypertension after mitral valve replacement. J Thorac Cardiovasc Surg 1985;89:567–72.

8. Said SI. Pulmonary metabolism of prostaglandins and vasoactive peptides. Annu Rev Physiol 1982; 44:257–68.

9. Lunn RJ. Inhaled nitric oxide therapy. Mayo Clin Proc 1995;70:247–55.

10. Christenson J, Lavoie A, O'Connor M, et al. The incidence and pathogenesis of cardiopulmonary deterioration after abrupt withdrawal of inhaled nitric oxide. Am J Respir Crit Care Med 2000;161:1443–9.

11. DeWet CJ, Affleck DG, Jacobsohn E, et al. Inhaled prostacyclin is safe, effective, and affordable in patients with pulmonary hypertension, right heart dysfunction, and refractory hypoxemia after cardiopulmonary surgery. J Thorac Cardiovasc Surg 2004;127:1058–67.

12. Lowson SM, Doctor A, Walsh BK, et al. Inhaled prostacyclin for the treatment of pulmonary hypertension after cardiac surgery. Crit Care Med 2002;30:2762–4.

13. Khan TA, Schnickel G, Ross D, et al. A prospective, randomized, crossover pilot study of inhaled nitric oxide versus inhaled prostacyclin in heart transplant and lung transplant recipients. J Thorac Cardiovasc Surg 2009;138:1417–24.

14. Santamore WP, Gray LA Jr. Left ventricular contributions to right ventricular systolic function during LVAD support. Ann Thorac Surg 1996;61:350–6.

15. Fukamachi K, McCarthy PM, Smedira NG, et al. Preoperative risk factors for right ventricular failure after implantable left ventricular assist device insertion. Ann Thorac Surg 1999;68:2181–4.

16. Goldstein JA, Vlahakes GJ, Verrier ED, et al. The role of right ventricular systolic dysfunction and elevated intrapericardial pressure on the genesis of low output in experimental right ventricular infarction. Circulation 1982;65:513–22.

Right Ventricular Failure in Patients with Left Ventricular Assist Devices

Jonathan D. Rich, MD

KEYWORDS

- Right ventricle • Ventricular assist device
- Left ventricular assist device
- Mechanical circulatory support • Heart failure • Treatment

According to the Interagency Registry for Mechanically Assisted Circulatory Support (INTERMACS) database, a registry of adult patients who receive durable Food and Drug Administration (FDA)-approved mechanical circulatory support (MCS) devices, nearly 4000 left ventricular assist devices (LVADs) have been implanted in the United States since June 2006, with more than one-third of these implants occurring in the past year alone.[1] It is speculated that the number of LVAD implants may increase at an even greater pace in the upcoming years given the increasing numbers of patients with advanced heart failure, the continued improvements occurring in LVAD technology, and with LVAD clinical trial designs beginning to target those with New York Heart Association Class III systolic heart failure (clinicaltrials.gov #NCT01452802 and clinicaltrials.gov #NCT01369407). Albeit a somewhat liberal and crude analysis, it has been suggested that nearly 300,000 current heart-failure patients could theoretically be justifiably targeted for LVAD consideration in the United States alone.[2] Although at present cardiac transplantation still remains the best long-term therapy for patients with end-stage heart failure, the reality is the vast majority of patients with advanced heart failure are either not suitable transplant candidates or will die on the transplant waiting list because of a shortage of available organs.[3] Thus, MCS with an LVAD frequently becomes the best alternative, viable therapeutic option for many of these patients short of palliative care and/or hospice.

LVAD therapy with the current generation of continuous-flow devices is indeed an increasingly attractive option for many patients with advanced heart failure because not only has it been shown to improve morbidity and mortality in comparison with optimal medical care, but it has even been proven to be superior to the previous generation of pulsatile LVADs.[4,5] Nevertheless, it also must be acknowledged that MCS with an LVAD remains short of a panacea, with many complications and challenges still occurring, and for which solutions are often far from satisfactory. One such complication is the development of right ventricular (RV) failure following the implant of an LVAD. While short-term right ventricular assist devices (RVADs) do exist, durable, long-term RVAD therapy currently remains unavailable in the United States, and RV failure after LVAD implant remains a highly relevant clinical problem. This article focuses on the epidemiology, mechanisms, and current management strategies of RV failure after LVAD implant in patients with advanced systolic heart failure who receive a continuous-flow LVAD.

Disclosures: The author has nothing to disclose.
Section of Cardiology, Department of Medicine, University of Chicago Medical Center, 5841 South Maryland Avenue, Chicago, IL 60637, USA
E-mail address: jrich@bsd.uchicago.edu

Cardiol Clin 30 (2012) 291–302
doi:10.1016/j.ccl.2012.03.008

EPIDEMIOLOGY

The most common cause of right-sided heart failure is left-sided heart failure.

—*Every medical school cardiovascular pathophysiology professor*

Because the above refrain has been ingrained in every medical school graduate ad nauseam, by logical extension one would surmise that the optimal treatment of RV failure should be the treatment of left ventricular (LV) failure. Thus, it may come as somewhat of a surprise to some that the persistence, worsening, or sometimes even new onset of RV failure after LVAD implant is anything but a trivial, uncommon scenario confronted by those who manage MCS patients. Although the reported incidence of RV failure after LVAD implant remains highly variable, a fair estimate is that approximately 15% to 25% of patients will suffer from RV failure following LVAD implant.[6–8] Reasons why the incidence of RV failure may vary widely in the published literature include differences in the type of LVAD studied (ie, pulsatile vs continuous flow), the nature and sizes of the patient populations enrolled in those studies, and the way in which RV failure is actually defined.

The most commonly used definition of post-LVAD RV failure in most studies, which closely approximates that defined by INTERMACS, is the presence of any one of the following: the need for postoperative intravenous inotropic support for longer than 14 days, the need for inhaled nitric oxide (NO) for longer than 48 hours, the need for right-sided MCS, and/or hospital discharge on an inotrope.[9] An alternative, though less commonly used definition of post-LVAD RV failure,[10] which more heavily emphasizes objective hemodynamic findings, is the presence of 2 or more of the following in the first 48 hours after LVAD implant and in the absence of cardiac tamponade: mean arterial pressure less than 55 mm Hg, central venous pressure greater than 16 mm Hg, mixed venous oxygen saturation less than 55%, cardiac index less than 2.0 L/min/m^2, and inotropic support greater than 20 units (according to the inotropic score[11]) (**Box 1**). Regardless of which definition is used, RV failure after LVAD implant has consistently been associated with worse clinical outcomes, including increased hospital length of stay,[6] worse end-organ function,[9] decreased bridge to transplant success,[9,12] and increased short-term and long-term mortality.[9,12,13] As a consequence, there have been considerable efforts to identify preoperative predictors of post-LVAD RV failure in an effort to reduce the incidence of this often devastating complication.

Box 1
Most commonly used definitions of acute RV failure after LVAD implant

1. The presence of any one of the following: the need for postoperative intravenous inotrope support for >14 days, the need for inhaled nitric oxide for >48 hours, the need for right-sided MCS, and/or hospital discharge on an inotrope

2. The presence of 2 or more of the following in the first 48 hours after LVAD implant in the absence of tamponade: mean arterial pressure <55 mm Hg, central venous pressure >16 mm Hg, mixed venous oxygen saturation <55%, cardiac index <2.0 L/min/m^2, inotropic support >20 units (according to the inotropic score)

CLINICAL PREDICTORS OF POST-LVAD RV FAILURE

It is easier to stay out than get out.
—*Mark Twain*

Because of the relatively high incidence of RV failure after LVAD implant and its deleterious impact on post-LVAD morbidity and mortality, many investigators have sought to identify preoperative risk factors predictive of post-LVAD RV failure. Although the majority of these investigations have been performed in the previous era of pulsatile LVADs, post-LVAD RV failure risk-assessment studies are beginning to emerge in patients receiving continuous-flow LVADs as well.[7,10,14–16] A summary of the major studies that have evaluated risk factors for post-LVAD RV failure, restricted to those studies that performed multivariate analyses, is shown in **Table 1**. A summary of those variables that appear most consistently across the many published studies are shown in **Box 2**.

Because of the retrospective nature of essentially all these studies, the differing definitions of RV failure used, and the substantial heterogeneity in the type of variables analyzed in each study, it is not unexpected that many of the studies have arrived at different conclusions. However, when examined closely, certain overlapping themes become apparent in terms of post-LVAD RV failure risk prediction. First, it seems that many of the same preoperative risk factors predisposing to worse overall post-LVAD outcomes are also risk factors for post-LVAD RV failure.[7,13,14,17–20] Thus, the "sicker" the patient is pre-LVAD implant, as reflected by those labeled as destination-therapy candidates only, those with evidence of

Table 1
Summary of key studies evaluating independent predictors of post-LVAD RV failure

Authors, Year	Device(s) Used	Sample Size (N)	Indication	RV Failure Definition	RV Failure Incidence (%)	Multivariate Predictors	Limitations
Ochiai et al,[68] 2002	A variety of pulsatile LVADs	245	97% as BTT	Need for an RVAD	9	Preoperative MCS; female sex; nonischemic etiology	Retrospective, almost all BTT patients, all pulsatile VADs, restricted RV failure definition
Dang et al,[9] 2006	Pulsatile Heartmate LVADs only	108	100% as BTT	RVAD; inotropes and/or vasodilators >14 d	39	Elevated intraoperative central venous pressure	Retrospective, all BTT, pulsatile VADs only
Fitzpatrick et al,[21] 2008	A wide variety of pulsatile LVADs 4% continuous-flow LVADs	266	Not defined	Need for an RVAD	37	Low RVSWI, low systolic BP; low cardiac index; severe preop. RV dysfunction by echo; previous sternotomy; elevated Cr	Retrospective, mostly pulsatile VADs, VAD indication not defined, unusually high incidence of RVAD
Matthews et al,[18] 2008	A wide variety of pulsatile LVADs 16% continuous-flow LVADs	197	94% as BTT	RVAD; inotropes >14 d or discharge on inotropes; NO >48 h	35	Preop. vasopressor use; AST >80; total bilirubin >2.0; Cr >2.3	Retrospective, majority pulsatile VADs, mostly BTT population
Patel et al,[14] 2008	56% pulsatile Heartmate XVE LVAD 44% continuous-flow Heartmate II LVAD	77	Not defined	RVAD or inotropic/vasodilator support for >14 d or both	38	Preop. IABP use	Retrospective, VAD indication not defined
Drakos et al,[13] 2010	A wide variety of pulsatile LVADs 14% continuous-flow LVADs	175	58% as BTT	RVAD; inotropes >14 d or discharge on inotropes; NO >48 h	44	Preop. IABP use; elevated PVR >2.8 Wood Units; DT as the indication; ACEI/ARB use	Retrospective, majority pulsatile VADs
Kormos et al,[7] 2010	Continuous-flow LVADs only	484	100% as BTT	RVAD or inotropic support >14 d and/or need to restart inotropes >14 d after implant	20	Preop. ventilator support, CVP/PCWP ratio >0.63; BUN >39 mg/dL	Retrospective, only BTT patients

Abbreviations: ACEI, angiotensin-converting enzyme inhibitor; ARB, angiotensin receptor blocker; AST, aspartate aminotransferase; BP, blood pressure; BTT, bridge to transplant; BUN, blood urea nitrogen; Cr, creatinine; CVP, central venous pressure; DT, destination therapy; IABP, intra-aortic balloon pumping; LVAD, left ventricular assist device; MCS, mechanical circulatory support; NO, nitric oxide; PCWP, pulmonary capillary wedge pressure; PVR, pulmonary vascular resistance; RV, right ventricular; RVAD, right ventricular assist device; RVSWI, right ventricular stroke work index; VAD, ventricular assist device.

significant end-organ dysfunction (ie, renal failure, hepatic dysfunction, and so forth), and those requiring the highest levels of preoperative hemodynamic support, including the need for mechanical ventilation, intravenous vasopressors, and/or an intra-aortic balloon pump (IABP) as a bridge to an LVAD, seem to identify those with the highest risk for post-LVAD RV failure. Second, and more specific to the status of the right ventricle itself, those patients with the highest right-sided filling pressures, particularly when accompanied by a low RV stroke work index, appear to be among the highest risk for post-LVAD RV failure (thus, those with RV failure pre-LVAD are more likely to suffer from RV failure post-LVAD implant).[6,7,9,21,22] In light of these risk factors, many have suggested that aggressive attempts to "tune up" patients before LVAD implant, including optimizing nutrition, coagulopathies, volume status, and so forth, might lower the incidence of post-LVAD RV failure; and although such recommendations certainly seem to be intuitive, whether such efforts will actually translate into improved outcomes for post-LVAD RV failure remains somewhat speculative.

RV PHYSIOLOGY AND PATHOPHYSIOLOGY AFTER LVAD IMPLANT

It ain't what you don't know that gets you into trouble. It's what you know for sure that just ain't so.

—Mark Twain

A brief review of basic RV physiology may help one to appreciate the challenges imposed on the

right ventricle as well as the observed variability in RV performance following an LVAD implant. Under normal conditions, whereas the left ventricle pumps into a high-pressure systemic circulation, the right ventricle pumps into a low-pressure pulmonary circulation. And whereas left coronary artery (and thus LV) perfusion occurs predominantly during diastole, right coronary artery perfusion occurs throughout the cardiac cycle, with approximately equal coronary flow occurring during systole and diastole. The interventricular septum is predominantly supplied by left coronary artery circulation, whereas the RV free wall receives its blood supply from RV marginal branches off the right coronary artery. The morphology and contractile patterns of the two ventricles are quite different as well. In contrast to the left ventricle, twisting and rotational movements do not contribute significantly to RV free wall contraction.[23] Finally, ventricular interdependence describes the concept that the structure and function of one ventricle directly affects the structure and function of the other ventricle.[24] From a simplistic perspective, the existence of ventricular interdependence can be explained by virtue of the fact that both ventricles share a common interventricular septum and both are encased by the surrounding pericardium. Adding an additional layer of anatomic complexity, both ventricles are also linked by spiral muscle bundles that encircle them in an interlacing fashion, thus forming a "highly interdependent functional unit."[25] Although diastolic ventricular interdependence is more readily appreciated in a variety of clinical contexts, both phases of the cardiac cycle are influenced by ventricular interdependence. Whereas diastolic ventricular interdependence is mediated through both the interventricular septum and the surrounding, intact pericardium, systolic ventricular interdependence seems to be mainly influenced by the interventricular septum.[24,26]

It is likely that a complex interplay among many of these factors and others contribute to changes in RV function occurring after an LVAD implant.[27] However, immediately following an LVAD implant, 3 rather dramatic physiologic changes occur that will strongly influence RV performance:

1. An increase in RV preload
2. A decrease in RV afterload
3. A change in RV contractility.

Given the important clinical consequences of these physiologic changes on RV function, a careful examination of each individually is warranted (**Fig. 1**).

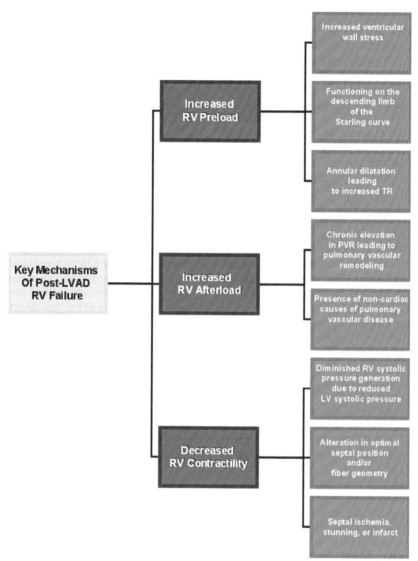

Fig. 1. Pathophysiology of post-LVAD RV failure. Although there are many contributory mechanisms to post-LVAD RV failure, 3 of the most significant include an increase in RV preload, a residual, increased RV afterload, and decreased RV contractility. Although RV afterload is expected to improve following LVAD, the time course of this resolution may vary. Also, if other causes of pulmonary vascular disease other than chronic heart failure are present, some degree of residual pulmonary hypertension may persist and contribute to RV dysfunction.

Increased RV Preload

The increase in venous return that occurs following LVAD implant is perhaps the simplest physiologic change to appreciate. The vast majority of patients before an LVAD implant are invariably in states of low cardiac output. For example, the mean cardiac index in the Randomized Evaluation of Mechanical Assistance for the Treatment of Congestive Heart Failure (REMATCH) trial was 1.9 ± 0.99 L/min/m^2.[4] Yet immediately following LVAD insertion, a near

doubling of left-sided resting cardiac output may occur in some patients.[20] Because the two ventricles are of course a single unit operating in series, this doubling of venous return places an immediate demand on the nonmechanically supported RV to accept this increased volume and in turn double its cardiac output. Moreover, the volume loading via blood transfusions and/or intravenous fluids that not uncommonly occurs in the intraoperative and postoperative settings may further exacerbate this demand imposed on the right ventricle. Finally, the increase in RV preload may cause further annular dilatation, leading to a worsening of the degree of tricuspid regurgitation (TR). Depending on the preoperative functional status of the right ventricle (and notwithstanding the acute, variable effects of cardiopulmonary bypass), this increase in venous return may pose an unacceptable demand on the right ventricle, which may result in acute RV failure. Thus, the common saying that the right ventricle is "preload dependent" is true after all—too much preload is deleterious!

Decreased RV Afterload

Chronic elevations in left ventricular end-diastolic pressure (LVEDP) result in secondary pulmonary hypertension (PH) and is the predominant mechanism whereby "left-sided heart failure causes right-sided heart failure." Thus, therapies that effectively unload the left ventricle and lower LVEDP will effectively also unload the right ventricle by lowering pulmonary artery (PA) pressures and by also attenuating the direct load imposed by the elevated LVEDP itself.[28] Because LVAD therapy is the most potent method of LV load reduction, one might logically deduce that an LVAD should also have a potently beneficial effect on RV function via RV afterload reduction and, indeed, this has been demonstrated by several studies.[27,29,30] This may in part explain why many studies have found elevated PA pressures to not be independently predictive of post-LVAD RV failure. Also, the vast majority of studies in the pulsatile era, and more recently in the continuous-flow LVAD era, have supported the observations that near complete resolution of PH will almost invariably occur after LVAD implant. In fact, even in those who meet criteria for having "fixed" PH pre-LVAD are likely to see resolution of the PH after LVAD implant.[31–33] These observations have in large part led to the common use of an LVAD as bridge to transplant in patients with severe PH, thus avoiding the risk of posttransplant RV failure. The one exception to the rule that near complete PH resolution will occur following LVAD therapy is when causes of PH other than those secondary to chronic LVEDP elevation coexist (ie, lung disease). In these instances, some degree of pulmonary vascular disease may persist, and thus a careful evaluation of comorbid cardiopulmonary conditions preoperatively is important. Although one can reliably predict PH resolution following LVAD implant, somewhat less predictable is the time course of the PH resolution (ranging from almost immediate to possibly weeks to months later) as well as the magnitude of impact that this unloading will have on RV function. Consider the following 3 common clinical scenarios:

Patient A: LVEDP 25 mm Hg, Mean PA pressure 30 mm Hg, Mean right atrial (RA) pressure 12 mm Hg, cardiac output 3.0 L/min.

Patient B: LVEDP 25 mm Hg, Mean PA pressure 40 mm Hg, Mean RA pressure 12 mm Hg, cardiac output 3.0 L/min.

Patient C: LVEDP 35 mm Hg, Mean PA pressure 40 mm Hg, Mean RA pressure 12 mm Hg, cardiac output 3.0 L/min.

Patient A has mild PH with a normal transpulmonary gradient (TPG), and LVAD therapy would be expected to result in fairly rapid resolution of the mild PH as the LVEDP is lowered. Although such afterload reduction is likely to be of benefit to the right ventricle, the overall net impact on RV function may only be modest when coupled with the increased venous return to the right ventricle with elevated preimplant filling pressures.

Patient B has moderate to severe PH with an elevated TPG in the setting of an elevated LVEDP. Assuming that the PH is the direct result of the chronic elevation in LVEDP, LVAD therapy should ultimately have a favorable and significant benefit on long-term RV function (not too dissimilar from the familiar clinical scenario of the patient with mitral stenosis associated with severe PH and RV dysfunction, whose PH resolves following mitral valve surgery[34]). However, because the time course of the PH resolution after LVAD implant may be variable, in the early postoperative period this patient may actually be at exceedingly high risk of acute RV failure.

Patient C also has moderate to severe PH but with a normal TPG in the face of a severely elevated LVEDP. As with patient B, LVAD therapy should ultimately result in significant RV afterload reduction, thus benefiting the right ventricle. However, 1 of 2 subsequent scenarios is possible. In one scenario the PH may resolve quickly in direct proportion to the LVEDP lowering, thus benefiting the right ventricle rather acutely. In the other scenario the possibility exists that following LVEDP lowering, an "unmasking" of pulmonary vascular disease might occur (with an increase in the calculated TPG), and thus this patient may respond in a more similar way to patient B.

These scenarios are intimately familiar to those who routinely perform vasodilator drug testing in the catheterization laboratory, and thus caution is needed when using resting pre-LVAD hemodynamics to predict the post-LVAD response. Although many studies emphasize low PA pressures to be a more ominous indicator of post-LVAD RV function (as a sign of severe RV pump dysfunction), it is also understandable why other studies have found the converse to be true. There may be an important role for preimplant drug testing during right heart catheterization to possibly predict (or to some extent simulate) the acute effects of LVAD therapy on PH and RV afterload, as well as the ability to evaluate RV reserve.[35]

Change in RV Contractility

Whereas the marked increase in RV preload (generally deleterious to the right ventricle) and the decrease in RV afterload (generally beneficial to the right ventricle) are, to variable extents, fairly predictable following LVAD implant, the net impact on overall RV performance may ultimately be determined through the complex changes mediated by ventricular interdependence. A deeper examination of the arrangement of the muscle fibers that comprise the right ventricle and left ventricle, respectively, provides further insight into the structure-function relationship already discussed. The RV free wall consists mostly of transverse myocardial fibers whereas the interventricular septal fibers are arranged in an oblique orientation, most closely resembling the LV free wall fiber configuration. Thus, although there exists no right-sided or left-sided septum per se, one could morphologically consider the septum to be more of an LV structure, than even a hybrid of both ventricles.[36] Nevertheless, there is no functional left-sided and right-sided septum; it functions as a single unit and affects the performance of both ventricles.[25] When the right ventricle contracts, the transverse fibers of the RV free wall constrict circumferentially in an inward fashion, while its longitudinal fibers shorten and draw the tricuspid annulus toward the apex. The oblique fibers of the interventricular septum, on the other hand, twist during contraction in similar fashion to the LV free wall, and serve to not only contribute to the pumping actions of the right ventricle but also provide traction for the RV free wall at its sites of attachment.[23,25] Because the inherent contractile strength of the oblique fibers of the interventricular septum are more powerful than the transverse fibers of the RV free wall, the septal contribution to RV stroke volume may be substantial.

As viewed through a series of fascinating animal studies, convincing evidence exists to support this concept that the left ventricle, mediated through the interventricular septum, contributes significantly to RV systolic performance.[37–41] Santamore and colleagues[39] performed a series of experiments using an isolated rabbit heart preparation. In one study, ligation of the anterior ventricular branches of the left coronary artery produced LV ischemia, which resulted in an almost immediate decrease in RV developed pressure. In a subsequent study,[38] the investigators vented the left ventricle (with similarities to an LVAD) and then subsequently cut out the LV free wall to nearly eliminate the LV contribution to RV pressure generation. Indeed, RV systolic pressure dropped dramatically but was subsequently reestablished when the LV free wall was resutured. When Hoffman and colleagues[40] performed a similar experiment but excised the RV free wall instead, replacing it with a xenograft pericardial patch, RV stroke volume was unaffected as long as LV systolic function was preserved. Specifically, they determined that LV contraction contributed 24% of LV stroke work to RV developed pressure, mediated via the interventricular septum which, interestingly, increased to 35% in the presence of PH. Finally, Goldstein and colleagues[41] performed a series of experiments in a canine RV free wall infarct model, also demonstrating the critical importance of septal function on RV stroke work.

The importance of the interventricular septum on RV performance has also been described in a variety of human conditions including congenital heart disease, RV dysplasia, RV infarct, and others.[25,42] It is therefore highly anticipated that following the implant of an LVAD, whereby the structure-function relationship between the right ventricle and left ventricle is instantly altered, these alterations in ventricular interdependence will undoubtedly affect the right ventricle in a critical way as well. For instance, the unloading effects of the LVAD results in a reduction in LV systolic pressure generation, which may in turn negatively affect RV developed pressure. Also, disruptions in the optimal fiber orientation of the septum and the relative distance of the septum to the RV free wall are likely to also affect RV function. Excessive septal bowing (either leftward or rightward) during LVAD therapy may stretch the septum in a way that distorts its normal architecture into a more transverse, less oblique fiber orientation, which may result in suboptimal contractile strength and RV dysfunction. Even small changes in the septum-RV free wall distance may cause large changes in volume displacement.[24,25] Finally, it is likely that both the functional status of the right ventricle at the time of LVAD implant as well as the presence and degree of PH are likely to influence the relative importance of the LV contribution to RV performance. Specifically, dependence on the septal contribution to RV function is likely to be greater in the setting of severe RV dysfunction and/or an elevated pulmonary vascular resistance (PVR).[24,25,43,44]

MANAGEMENT

When a lot of remedies are suggested for a disease, that means it cannot be cured.

—Anton Chekhov

The approach to managing post-LVAD RV failure can be conveniently organized into 3 distinct time periods: preoperative, intraoperative, and postoperative.

Preoperative Management

When possible, LVAD implants should generally be delayed until several, often reversible, medical problems can be adequately addressed. First, decompensated RV failure should be aggressively managed when possible before LVAD implant, with a particular emphasis on aggressive diuresis and the use of systemic vasodilators to lower PA pressures and achieve a near normal RA pressure. The use of direct pulmonary artery vasodilators, however, should not be routinely used in the pre-LVAD setting because of the risk of pulmonary edema.[45,46] In addition to interventions specific to the right ventricle, it is of the essence that systemic problems including malnutrition, coagulopathies, acute end-organ dysfunction, and other metabolic derangements be optimized as well.[17]

If following a thorough preoperative assessment the patient is deemed to be at high risk for post-LVAD RV failure, strong consideration should be given to the use of early (albeit temporary) mechanical RV support. Although randomized studies are lacking, several observational studies have suggested that clinical outcomes are improved with early, planned biventricular support with an RVAD compared with those patients who are returned to the operating room for a delayed RVAD implant.[47] The actual decision to implant an RVAD in the high-risk patient could be made in the preoperative setting. Alternatively, and as is more often the case, the decision could be made intraoperatively, guided by the use of both invasive hemodynamic monitoring and transesophageal echocardiography (TEE) at the time of weaning from cardiopulmonary bypass. Generally speaking, if favorable hemodynamics are not achieved within a reasonable amount of time or if multiple high-dose inotropes are required to achieve hemodynamic stability, strong consideration should be given for temporary RVAD placement.[48] Although many short-term RVADs are available, the Centrimag (Levitronix, Waltham, MA, USA) device is most commonly used at the author's institution.[49]

Intraoperative Management

A frequently encountered decision that must be made at the time of LVAD implant is whether to repair (or occasionally replace) the tricuspid valve in the presence of significant TR. Although some studies have shown severe preoperative TR to be a risk factor for post-LVAD RV failure,[16,50] equipoise exists regarding whether actually intervening on the tricuspid valve at the time of LVAD implant will result in less post-LVAD RV failure and/or improved clinical outcomes. Indeed, reasonable arguments can be made on both sides. Because in the vast majority of cases the TR is secondary to the abnormal loading conditions that result in RV dysfunction and tricuspid annular dilatation, some argue that over time the TR will inevitably lessen as adequate unloading occurs with the LVAD, and indeed several studies support this contention.[51,52] Others, however, have argued that the increased RV preload that occurs after LVAD implant, coupled with architectural changes that may include a leftward shift of the interventricular septum with restriction of the septal leaflet of the tricuspid valve, will not result in reliable improvements in TR after LVAD implant and thus surgical correction is indicated. Recently, Piacentino and colleagues[53] demonstrated that in patients with moderate or severe TR, concomitant tricuspid valve repair resulted in a shorter duration of postoperative inotropes and hospital length of stay, with a trend toward improved survival, compared with the cohort without a tricuspid intervention. At the authors' institution, tricuspid valve repair at the time of LVAD implant in the presence of at least moderate TR is favored. A prospective clinical trial to address this important question is warranted, as the existing data addressing this question are all retrospective and nonrandomized.

Another commonly encountered surgical consideration is the approach to obstructive coronary artery disease at the time of LVAD implant. The 2 contexts in which strong consideration should be given to concomitant bypass surgery are in the presence of proximal to mid left anterior descending artery (LAD) disease and proximal right coronary artery (RCA) disease, respectively. Regarding the LAD, in addition to supplying the anterior wall of the left ventricle, the bigger concern may be the risk of septal ischemia or septal infarct, thus losing the septal contribution to RV function after LVAD implant.[54] With regard to the RCA, the major concern is the risk that RCA ischemia or an RV infarct could compromise the RV marginal branches off the dominant RCA, which supply the RV free wall. Although percutaneous revascularization before or following LVAD implant could be considered, the need for dual antiplatelet therapy in addition to standard LVAD anticoagulation makes this option somewhat less attractive.

Immediately following the LVAD implant, the LVAD should be turned on and initial LVAD speeds should be adjusted gradually to achieve an appropriate balance between adequate LV unloading with sufficient ventricular assist device (VAD) flows, but not at the expense of excessive leftward septal bowing. The use of TEE and invasive hemodynamic monitoring are thus essential components of initiating LVAD support. Emerging from the operating room at somewhat lower initial LVAD speeds may be of particular importance in the patient at increased risk of post-LVAD RV failure, where an initial strategy of "partial" LV unloading may be preferable to higher speeds in order to avoid excessive RV preload and leftward septal bowing, which may worsen RV function in the already dysfunctional and perhaps stunned RV following cardiopulmonary bypass.[55]

Postoperative Management

Following the vast majority of LVAD implants, inotropic RV support will be required and should be initiated in the operating room before or simultaneous to weaning of cardiopulmonary bypass. The exact choice of inotrope (ie, dobutamine vs milrinone vs other) is not likely to be of great significance. Although milrinone is an inotrope that also possesses potent vasodilatory properties, in contrast to popular belief, the notion that milrinone is preferable to dobutamine because of its selective pulmonary artery vasodilatory properties is largely unfounded.[56,57] The rate at which the inotropic agents should be weaned is likely to be highly variable and patient specific. Close monitoring of RA pressures is of utmost importance, with consideration for early use of diuretics, particularly in the setting of ongoing bleeding whereby it is anticipated that excessive volume loading may occur because of the need to infuse multiple blood products. Also, because RV stroke volume may be significantly impaired in the early postoperative period, maintenance of sinus rhythm and sustaining an adequate heart rate are both necessary to maintain a sufficient RV cardiac output. In the setting of relative chronotropic incompetence, atrial pacing at approximately 100 beats per minute should be considered.

In the face of an elevated PVR and/or manifestations of early signs of RV dysfunction, the use of direct pulmonary artery vasodilators such as inhaled NO or inhaled prostacyclin are often used. The use of inhaled NO following LVAD implant gained momentum following the publication of a small double-blind, randomized study, which showed that the use of inhaled NO following cardiopulmonary bypass wean led to significant reductions in mean PA pressures and increases in LVAD flows compared with inhaled nitrogen.[58] However, though inhaled NO has subsequently

and consistently been shown to effectively lower PA pressures in other studies as well, its impact on RV failure and other clinical outcomes remains uncertain.[59,60] Recently, Potapov and colleagues[60] published the results of a prospective, randomized, double-blind, multicenter, placebo-controlled trial of inhaled NO immediately after LVAD implant in patients with an elevated PVR (≥2.5 Wood units). The study failed to show a reduction in post-LVAD RV failure, though its final interpretation may be limited by the high crossover rate and the unconventional definition of RV failure used in the study. Despite the neutral findings in this study, the author continues to have a low threshold for using inhaled NO in patients with a markedly elevated PVR and/or early signs of acute RV failure.

In LVAD patients who have a significantly elevated PVR that does not improve in the early postoperative days, particularly in those with significant, concomitant RV dysfunction, use of an oral phosphodiesterase type 5A inhibitor is a reasonable therapeutic strategy. Tedford and colleagues[61] compared the use of oral sildenafil in patients with a persistently elevated PVR (>3 Wood units) at 1 to 2 weeks post-VAD implant with a historical control cohort that did not receive sildenafil. At approximately 3 to 4 months after VAD implant, patients receiving sildenafil had significantly lower mean PA pressures and PVR compared with those who did not receive sildenafil. In addition to its ability to lower PA pressures, sildenafil may also provide pleiotropic benefits via increasing RV contractility.[62] However, it should be noted that even in those not receiving sildenafil in this study, dramatic reductions in PVR eventually occurred, highlighting the potent ability of LV unloading to reverse PH.

SUMMARY AND FUTURE DIRECTIONS

This article reviewed the epidemiology, predictors, mechanisms, and management strategies of patients with post-LVAD RV failure, particularly RV failure occurring early after LVAD implant. However, it must be emphasized that there is a conspicuous paucity of data surrounding RV failure occurring "later" after LVAD implant, and this is far from a trivial point. Many LVAD patients may ultimately be limited by RV dysfunction despite excellent LVAD function and LV unloading. It can even be argued, particularly as it relates specifically to those patients who receive an LVAD as destination therapy, that it is RV failure that develops and persists later after LVAD implantation that is most relevant, whereby exercise capacity and quality of life (in addition to mortality) may be greatly affected.[63] While it may be speculated that intermediate and late post-LVAD RV failure share many of the same predictors, mechanisms, and management strategies as those in the early post-LVAD phase, significant differences undoubtedly exist as well.[15] In fact, whereas favorable cellular and molecular signatures of reverse remodeling and function clearly occur in the left ventricle following LVAD implant, the same favorable changes may not be occurring in the right ventricle.[64–66] Although progress is being made toward the development and use of permanent RVAD and bilateral VAD systems, the assessment and management of the right ventricle in the majority patients with LV failure who receive an LVAD is likely to remain a critical issue for many years to come.[67]

REFERENCES

1. Interagency Registry for Mechanically Assisted Circulatory Support (INTERMACS) Quarterly Statistical Summary Report. The Data Collection and Analysis Center at the University of Alabama at Birmingham. 2011.
2. Starling RC, Gorodeski EZ. Potential population for long-term use of left ventricular assist devices. In: Kormos RL, Miller LW, editors. Mechanical circulatory support: a companion to Braunwald's heart disease. Philadelphia (PA): Elsevier; 2011. p. 11–21.
3. Taylor DO, Stehlik J, Edwards LB, et al. Registry of the international society for heart and lung transplantation: twenty-sixth official adult heart transplant report—2009. J Heart Lung Transplant 2009;28(10): 1007–22.
4. Rose EA, Gelijns AC, Moskowitz AJ, et al. Long-term use of a left ventricular assist device for end-stage heart failure. N Engl J Med 2001;345(20):1435–43.
5. Slaughter MS, Rogers JG, Milano CA, et al. Advanced heart failure treated with continuous-flow left ventricular assist device. N Engl J Med 2009; 361(23):2241–51.
6. Kavarana MN, Pessin-Minsley MS, Urtecho J, et al. Right ventricular dysfunction and organ failure in left ventricular assist device recipients: a continuing problem. Ann Thorac Surg 2002;73(3):745–50.
7. Kormos RL, Teuteberg JJ, Pagani FD, et al. Right ventricular failure in patients with the HeartMate II continuous-flow left ventricular assist device: incidence, risk factors, and effect on outcomes. J Thorac Cardiovasc Surg 2010;139(5):1316–24.
8. Genovese EA, Dew MA, Teuteberg JJ, et al. Incidence and patterns of adverse event onset during the first 60 days after ventricular assist device implantation. Ann Thorac Surg 2009;88(4): 1162–70.
9. Dang NC, Topkara VK, Mercando M, et al. Right heart failure after left ventricular assist device implantation in patients with chronic congestive heart failure. J Heart Lung Transplant 2006;25(1):1–6.
10. Kukucka M, Stepanenko A, Potapov E, et al. Right-to-left ventricular end-diastolic diameter ratio and prediction of right ventricular failure with continuous-flow left ventricular assist devices. J Heart Lung Transplant 2011;30(1):64–9.
11. Kormos RL, Gasior TA, Kawai A, et al. Transplant candidate's clinical status rather than right ventricular function defines need for univentricular versus biventricular support. J Thorac Cardiovasc Surg 1996;111(4):773–82 [discussion: 782–3].
12. Morgan JA, John R, Lee BJ, et al. Is severe right ventricular failure in left ventricular assist device recipients a risk factor for unsuccessful bridging to transplant and post-transplant mortality. Ann Thorac Surg 2004;77(3):859–63.
13. Drakos SG, Janicki L, Horne BD, et al. Risk factors predictive of right ventricular failure after left ventricular assist device implantation. Am J Cardiol 2010; 105(7):1030–5.
14. Patel ND, Weiss ES, Schaffer J, et al. Right heart dysfunction after left ventricular assist device implantation: a comparison of the pulsatile HeartMate I and axial-flow HeartMate II devices. Ann Thorac Surg 2008;86(3):832–40 [discussion: 832–40].
15. Baumwol J, Macdonald PS, Keogh AM, et al. Right heart failure and "failure to thrive" after left ventricular assist device: clinical predictors and outcomes. J Heart Lung Transplant 2011;30(8):888–95.
16. Potapov EV, Stepanenko A, Dandel M, et al. Tricuspid incompetence and geometry of the right ventricle as predictors of right ventricular function after implantation of a left ventricular assist device. J Heart Lung Transplant 2008;27(12):1275–81.
17. Lietz K, Long JW, Kfoury AG, et al. Outcomes of left ventricular assist device implantation as destination therapy in the post-REMATCH era: implications for patient selection. Circulation 2007;116(5): 497–505.
18. Matthews JC, Koelling TM, Pagani FD, et al. The right ventricular failure risk score a pre-operative tool for assessing the risk of right ventricular failure in left ventricular assist device candidates. J Am Coll Cardiol 2008;51(22):2163–72.
19. Santambrogio L, Bianchi T, Fuardo M, et al. Right ventricular failure after left ventricular assist device insertion: preoperative risk factors. Interact Cardiovasc Thorac Surg 2006;5(4):379–82.
20. Farrar DJ, Hill JD, Pennington DG, et al. Preoperative and postoperative comparison of patients with univentricular and biventricular support with the Thoratec ventricular assist device as a bridge to cardiac transplantation. J Thorac Cardiovasc Surg 1997;113(1):202–9.

21. Fitzpatrick JR 3rd, Frederick JR, Hsu VM, et al. Risk score derived from pre-operative data analysis predicts the need for biventricular mechanical circulatory support. J Heart Lung Transplant 2008;27(12): 1286–92.

22. Fukamachi K, McCarthy PM, Smedira NG, et al. Preoperative risk factors for right ventricular failure after implantable left ventricular assist device insertion. Ann Thorac Surg 1999;68(6):2181–4.

23. Haddad F, Hunt SA, Rosenthal DN, et al. Right ventricular function in cardiovascular disease, part I: anatomy, physiology, aging, and functional assessment of the right ventricle. Circulation 2008;117(11): 1436–48.

24. Santamore WP, Dell'Italia LJ. Ventricular interdependence: significant left ventricular contributions to right ventricular systolic function. Prog Cardiovasc Dis 1998;40(4):289–308.

25. Saleh S, Liakopoulos OJ, Buckberg GD. The septal motor of biventricular function. Eur J Cardiothorac Surg 2006;29(Suppl 1):S126–38.

26. Janicki JS, Weber KT. The pericardium and ventricular interaction, distensibility, and function. Am J Physiol 1980;238(4):H494–503.

27. Farrar DJ, Compton PG, Hershon JJ, et al. Right heart interaction with the mechanically assisted left heart. World J Surg 1985;9(1):89–102.

28. Tedford RJ, Hassoun PM, Mathai SC, et al. Pulmonary capillary wedge pressure augments right ventricular pulsatile loading. Circulation 2012;125(2):289–97.

29. Farrar DJ, Compton PG, Dajee H, et al. Right heart function during left heart assist and the effects of volume loading in a canine preparation. Circulation 1984;70(4):708–16.

30. Morita S, Kormos RL, Mandarino WA, et al. Right ventricular/arterial coupling in the patient with left ventricular assistance. Circulation 1992;86(Suppl 5): II316–25.

31. John R, Liao K, Kamdar F, et al. Effects on pre- and posttransplant pulmonary hemodynamics in patients with continuous-flow left ventricular assist devices. J Thorac Cardiovasc Surg 2010;140(2):447–52.

32. Alba AC, Rao V, Ross HJ, et al. Impact of fixed pulmonary hypertension on post-heart transplant outcomes in bridge-to-transplant patients. J Heart Lung Transplant 2010;29(11):1253–8.

33. Etz CD, Welp HA, Tjan TD, et al. Medically refractory pulmonary hypertension: treatment with nonpulsatile left ventricular assist devices. Ann Thorac Surg 2007;83(5):1697–705.

34. Zener JC, Hancock EW, Shumway NE, et al. Regression of extreme pulmonary hypertension after mitral valve surgery. Am J Cardiol 1972;30(8):820–6.

35. Deswarte G, Kirsch M, Lesault PF, et al. Right ventricular reserve and outcome after continuous-flow left ventricular assist device implantation. J Heart Lung Transplant 2010;29(10):1196–8.

36. Weber KT, Janicki JS, Shroff S, et al. Contractile mechanics and interaction of the right and left ventricles. Am J Cardiol 1981;47(3):686–95.

37. Damiano RJ Jr, La Follette P Jr, Cox JL, et al. Significant left ventricular contribution to right ventricular systolic function. Am J Physiol 1991;261(5 Pt 2): H1514–24.

38. Li KS, Santamore WP. Contribution of each wall to biventricular function. Cardiovasc Res 1993;27(5): 792–800.

39. Santamore WP, Lynch PR, Heckman JL, et al. Left ventricular effects on right ventricular developed pressure. J Appl Physiol 1976;41(6):925–30.

40. Hoffman D, Sisto D, Frater RW, et al. Left-to-right ventricular interaction with a noncontracting right ventricle. J Thorac Cardiovasc Surg 1994;107(6): 1496–502.

41. Goldstein JA, Tweddell JS, Barzilai B, et al. Importance of left ventricular function and systolic ventricular interaction to right ventricular performance during acute right heart ischemia. J Am Coll Cardiol 1992;19(3):704–11.

42. Dibble CT, Lima JA, Bluemke DA, et al. Regional left ventricular systolic function and the right ventricle: the multi-ethnic study of atherosclerosis right ventricle study. Chest 2011;140(2):310–6.

43. Farrar DJ. Physiology of ventricular interactions during ventricular assistance. Armonk (NY): Futura Publishing Co, Inc; 2000.

44. Klima UP, Lee MY, Guerrero JL, et al. Determinants of maximal right ventricular function: role of septal shift. J Thorac Cardiovasc Surg 2002;123(1):72–80.

45. Bocchi EA, Bacal F, Auler Junior JO, et al. Inhaled nitric oxide leading to pulmonary edema in stable severe heart failure. Am J Cardiol 1994;74(1):70–2.

46. Dickstein ML, Burkhoff D. A theoretic analysis of the effect of pulmonary vasodilation on pulmonary venous pressure: implications for inhaled nitric oxide therapy. J Heart Lung Transplant 1996;15(7): 715–21.

47. Fitzpatrick JR 3rd, Frederick JR, Hiesinger W, et al. Early planned institution of biventricular mechanical circulatory support results in improved outcomes compared with delayed conversion of a left ventricular assist device to a biventricular assist device. J Thorac Cardiovasc Surg 2009;137(4):971–7.

48. Loforte A, Montalto A, Lilla Della Monica P, et al. Simultaneous temporary CentriMag right ventricular assist device placement in HeartMate II left ventricular assist system recipients at high risk of right ventricular failure. Interact Cardiovasc Thorac Surg 2010;10(6):847–50.

49. Bhama JK, Kormos RL, Toyoda Y, et al. Clinical experience using the Levitronix CentriMag system for temporary right ventricular mechanical circulatory support. J Heart Lung Transplant 2009;28(9): 971–6.

50. Puwanant S, Hamilton KK, Klodell CT, et al. Tricuspid annular motion as a predictor of severe right ventricular failure after left ventricular assist device implantation. J Heart Lung Transplant 2008;27(10):1102–7.

51. Lee S, Kamdar F, Madlon-Kay R, et al. Effects of the HeartMate II continuous-flow left ventricular assist device on right ventricular function. J Heart Lung Transplant 2010;29(2):209–15.

52. Saeed D, Kidambi T, Shalli S, et al. Tricuspid valve repair with left ventricular assist device implantation: is it warranted? J Heart Lung Transplant 2011;30(5):530–5.

53. Piacentino V 3rd, Troupes CD, Ganapathi AM, et al. Clinical impact of concomitant tricuspid valve procedures during left ventricular assist device implantation. Ann Thorac Surg 2011;92(4):1414–8 [discussion: 1418–9].

54. Daly RC, Chandrasekaran K, Cavarocchi NC, et al. Ischemia of the interventricular septum. A mechanism of right ventricular failure during mechanical left ventricular assist. J Thorac Cardiovasc Surg 1992;103(6):1186–91.

55. Pegg TJ, Selvanayagam JB, Karamitsos TD, et al. Effects of off-pump versus on-pump coronary artery bypass grafting on early and late right ventricular function. Circulation 2008;117(17):2202–10.

56. Feneck RO, Sherry KM, Withington PS, et al. Comparison of the hemodynamic effects of milrinone with dobutamine in patients after cardiac surgery. J Cardiothorac Vasc Anesth 2001;15(3):306–15.

57. Packer M. Vasodilator therapy for primary pulmonary hypertension. Limitations and hazards. Ann Intern Med 1985;103(2):258–70.

58. Argenziano M, Choudhri AF, Moazami N, et al. Randomized, double-blind trial of inhaled nitric oxide in LVAD recipients with pulmonary hypertension. Ann Thorac Surg 1998;65(2):340–5.

59. Kukucka M, Potapov E, Stepanenko A, et al. Acute impact of left ventricular unloading by left ventricular assist device on the right ventricle geometry and function: effect of nitric oxide inhalation. J Thorac Cardiovasc Surg 2011;141(4):1009–14.

60. Potapov E, Meyer D, Swaminathan M, et al. Inhaled nitric oxide after left ventricular assist device implantation: a prospective, randomized, double-blind, multicenter, placebo-controlled trial. J Heart Lung Transplant 2011;30(8):870–8.

61. Tedford RJ, Hemnes AR, Russell SD, et al. PDE5A inhibitor treatment of persistent pulmonary hypertension after mechanical circulatory support. Circ Heart Fail 2008;1(4):213–9.

62. Nagendran J, Archer SL, Soliman D, et al. Phosphodiesterase type 5 is highly expressed in the hypertrophied human right ventricle, and acute inhibition of phosphodiesterase type 5 improves contractility. Circulation 2007;116(3):238–48.

63. Di Salvo TG, Mathier M, Semigran MJ, et al. Preserved right ventricular ejection fraction predicts exercise capacity and survival in advanced heart failure. J Am Coll Cardiol 1995;25(5):1143–53.

64. Barbone A, Holmes JW, Heerdt PM, et al. Comparison of right and left ventricular responses to left ventricular assist device support in patients with severe heart failure: a primary role of mechanical unloading underlying reverse remodeling. Circulation 2001;104(6):670–5.

65. Maeder MT, Leet A, Ross A, et al. Changes in right ventricular function during continuous-flow left ventricular assist device support [corrected]. J Heart Lung Transplant 2009;28(4):360–6.

66. Palardy M, Nohria A, Rivero J, et al. Right ventricular dysfunction during intensive pharmacologic unloading persists after mechanical unloading. J Card Fail 2010;16(3):218–24.

67. Loforte A, Monica PL, Montalto A, et al. HeartWare third-generation implantable continuous flow pump as biventricular support: mid-term follow-up. Interact Cardiovasc Thorac Surg 2011;12(3):458–60.

68. Ochiai Y, McCarthy PM, Smedira NG, et al. Predictors of severe right ventricular failure after implantable left ventricular assist device insertion: analysis of 245 patients. Circulation 2002;106(12 Suppl 1):I198–202.

Percutaneous Mechanical Support for the Failing Right Heart

James A. Goldstein, MD[a],*, Morton J. Kern, MD[b]

KEYWORDS

- Percutaneous mechanical support • Right heart failure
- Inferior myocardial infarction • Ventricular assist device

Hemodynamically severe right ventricular (RV) failure is an increasingly common clinical problem resulting from one or more of several different pathophysiologic mechanisms. Severe RV failure complicates primary cardiomyopathic conditions, including acute RV infarction (RVI) associated with transmural ST elevation inferior myocardial infarction (IMI) and severe chronic decompensated congestive heart failure (CHF). Profound RV failure also may result from primary increased afterload, either acutely in patients with massive or submassive acute pulmonary embolism, or in the setting of chronic pulmonary hypertension of any origin. RV failure also complicates congenital heart lesions. Finally, RV failure is a feared and potentially lethal complication following cardiac surgery, including any case after cardiopulmonary bypass, following transplantation, and (increasingly) after surgical left ventricular assist device (LVAD) placement.

In contrast to severe left ventricular (LV) failure, RV failure is typically more reversible—a disparate response attributable to dramatic differences between the ventricles with respect to structure, loading conditions, metabolism, and oxygen supply-demand characteristics. Regardless of the clinical scenario, severe RV failure may result in profound hemodynamic compromise and increased mortality. This article considers the available mechanical approaches to provide hemodynamic support to treat profound RV failure in the common clinical scenarios in which percutaneous mechanical RV support may be most beneficial.

CLINICAL SCENARIOS REQUIRING RV MECHANICAL SUPPORT

Acute RVI

Nearly 50% of patients with acute ST elevation IMI suffer concomitant RVI, which is associated with higher in-hospital morbidity and mortality related to hemodynamic and electrophysiologic complications.[1,2] Although most RVI cases respond promptly and dramatically to successful primary percutaneous revascularization with recovery of RV function, less hemodynamic compromise, and excellent clinical outcome,[2] some patients experience refractory shock. Given that the ischemic RV nearly always recovers over time (if the patient can survive the acute hemodynamic compromise), temporary mechanical hemodynamic support may provide a bridge-to-recovery.[3,4] Anecdotally, intra-aortic balloon pumping (IABP) may be beneficial in such cases, though there is little research to shed light on the mechanisms by which IABP exerts salutary effects in acute RV shock. It is unlikely that IABP directly improves RV performance but, instead, it functions by stabilizing mean aortic pressure, thereby improving coronary perfusion pressure in severely hypotensive patients. Because RV myocardial blood flow depends on perfusion

[a] Department of Cardiovascular Medicine, Beaumont Health System, 3601 West 13 Mile Road, Royal Oak, MI 48073, USA; [b] Department of Cardiology, Long Beach VA Hospital, 5901 East 7th Street, 3rd, Long Beach, CA 90822, USA
* Corresponding author.
E-mail address: JGOLDSTEIN@beaumont.edu

Cardiol Clin 30 (2012) 303–310
doi:10.1016/j.ccl.2012.03.007
0733-8651/12/$ – see front matter © 2012 Published by Elsevier Inc.

pressure, IABP augmentation of RV perfusion could benefit RV function, particularly if the right coronary artery has been recanalized or if there is collateral supply to an occluded vessel. IABP may also potentially improve LV performance in those patients with hypotension and concomitant depressed LV function. Because performance of the dysfunctional RV is largely dependent on LV-septal contraction,[1,2] RV performance may also benefit.

In RVI shock cases refractory to IABP, temporary mechanical support with a VAD may be lifesaving. Given the anticipation of ultimate and usually short-term RV recovery in these patients, a percutaneous VAD is preferable to surgical implantation. Recent reports suggest that percutaneous a right VAD (RVAD) can improve hemodynamics in RVI patients with refractory life-threatening low output, thereby providing the reperfused RV a bridge to recovery.

Severe Pulmonary Hypertension

Right heart failure (RHF) attributable to severe pulmonary hypertension is a life-threatening condition, whether due to acute elevated pulmonary resistance resulting from massive and submassive pulmonary embolus or owing to chronic pulmonary vascular changes. Regardless of the setting, RV failure is an ominous hemodynamic problem. Unfortunately, there is little data to guide insight as to whether RVAD mechanical support might be effective in this scenario. On the one hand, it could be argued that mechanical support of RV failure attributable to primary increased afterload will not improve RV output through fixed resistance. However, mechanical support could beneficially unload the failing RV and give it sufficient "rest" while seeking definitive or palliative interventions aimed at reducing pulmonary resistance by pharmacologic pulmonary vasodilatation and/or thrombectomy (mechanical or surgical).

RV Failure in Chronic Decompensated Heart Failure

RV failure commonly complicates chronic decompensated congestive heart failure. The presence and severity of RV failure correlates with increased morbidity and mortality in patients with CHF.[5,6] RV failure is a particularly feared complication in patients undergoing LVAD therapy.[7–10] It occurs in up to 25% of cases, is associated with worse clinical outcome, and (in some cases) necessitates temporary RVAD support. An RV failure risk score, employing preoperative clinical, laboratory, ECG, and hemodynamic parameters, effectively stratifies the risk of RV failure and death after LVAD implantation.[10]

Postsurgical RV Failure

Isolated RHF after cardiac surgery is uncommon but the prognosis is poor.[11–15] Postcardiotomy RHF can be caused by prolonged cardioplegic arrest, inadequate myocardial protection, and right coronary occlusion due to coronary vasospasm, air embolization, and thrombus. Management for these patients is challenging and mortality may exceed 50%; however, RVADs may improve these outcomes.

Mechanical Interventions and Support Devices for RV Failure

Mechanical approaches to RV failure are designed to improve transpulmonary delivery of LV preload and to unload the failing RV. Mechanical interventions include atrial septostomy, balloon catheter counterpulsation, and direct mechanical hemodynamic support devices (surgically and percutaneously implanted).

Atrial septostomy

Atrial septostomy was the earliest mechanical approach to RV failure. Initially performed surgically and later percutaneously, the "Rashkind" balloon atrial septostomy[16] is primarily used to treat life-threatening cyanotic congenital heart defects in infants (typically, dextrotransposition of the great arteries). The technique involves the use of a balloon-tipped catheter without end holes that is passed through the atrial septum via transseptal puncture. Once the balloon catheter is on the left atrial side of the septum, the balloon is inflated and it is forcibly retracted through the septum to create a hole, permitting right atrial pressure and flow to move into the left atrium, functionally decompressing the elevated right heart pressures. It has seen limited use as palliation for end-stage pulmonary hypertension and it has been rarely employed for refractory shock in patients with acute RVI. This intervention improves systemic blood flow and unloads the failing dilated RV; however, this is at the cost of severe hypoxemia attributable to the intentionally created right-to-left shunt.

IABP

IABP supports the failing LV by diastolic augmentation and systolic unloading. IABP may help stabilize blood pressure in patients with acute RV infarction and shock. Although the mechanisms have not been delineated, IABP benefits are presumably mediated by augmenting mean aortic pressure, which augments LV performance, systemic perfusion, and coronary blood flow. Given these mechanisms, it is not surprising that mechanical assistance employing balloon counterpulsation in the pulmonary artery has been disappointing. This intervention cannot improve RV perfusion and has very limited capacity to reduce afterload or lower pulmonary resistance.

RVAD Devices

The standard approach to RV mechanical support is a surgically implantable RVAD, which is adapted from standard intermediate to long-term LVAD technology (**Fig. 1**) used for acute support. Destination LVADs have become accepted as a valuable therapy for end-stage heart failure during recent years.[17–21] This is mainly a result of miniaturization and increased reliability of the available devices, improvement of both patient selection and perioperative management, and a significant decline in adverse event rates associated with the use of LVADs. Important consideration for VADs in general include flow and pressure characteristics, shear stress, size of the pump, adaptability to diverse applications and patient requirements, rapid and easy deployment, blood exposure times to artificial surfaces, hemolysis and thrombogenicity, as well as device durability and costs.

Isolated RVADs were first used for postcardiotomy RV failure. In a series of 30 patients requiring isolated RVAD support, 43% survived to device explant, with significant RV recovery.[14] In more recent reports concerning use of a centrifugal device for univentricular or biventricular failure, 30 day survival was 30%.[21] In patients with severe decompensated LV failure, there is a growing use of mechanical circulatory support employing surgically implantable VADs, used for bridge-to-recovery, bridge-to-transplant, and primary destination therapy.[17–20] In a series of 100 consecutive acute myocardial infarction cardiogenic shock

patients supported with the AB5000 Ventricle device (Abiomed Inc, Danvers, MA, USA) 8% of the patients were RVAD only. Of the 40% of the patients who survived to discharge, 64% were discharged after myocardial recovery had occurred.[22] The development of RV failure is a feared complication of LVAD insertion for decompensated cardiomyopathy and RVAD support is now most commonly applied in patients also undergoing LVAD support, either primarily at the time of LVAD implant or in those in whom RV failure develops post-LVAD implantation.[7–10,17] Kormos and colleagues[18] evaluated the incidence, risk factors, and effect on outcomes of RV failure in 484 patients implanted with continuous-flow LVADs treated with the HeartMate II LVAD (Thoratec, Pleasanton, CA, USA). In this bridge-to-transplantation clinical trial, patients were examined for the occurrence of RV failure, defined as requiring an RVAD, 14 or more days of inotropic support after implantation, and/or inotropic support starting more than 14 days after LVAD implantation. Overall, 30 (6%) patients receiving LVADs required an RVAD, 35 (7%) required extended inotropes, and 33 (7%) required late inotropes. A significantly greater percentage of patients without RV failure survived to transplantation, recovery, or ongoing device support at 180 days compared with patients with RV failure (89% vs 71%, P<.001). This study demonstrated that the incidence of RV failure in patients with a HeartMate II VAD is comparable or less than that of patients with pulsatile-flow devices and that RV failure portends significantly worse outcomes. Patients at risk for RV failure might benefit from preoperative optimization of right heart function or planned biventricular support.

For long-term biventricular support, there are several options.[20,23] One approach is implantation of two pulsatile displacement pumps, which requires either an extensive operation with the creation of large pockets in the abdominal

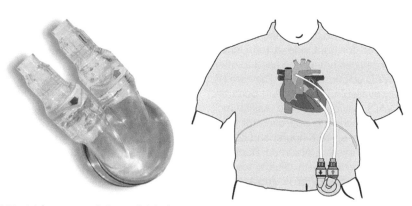

Fig. 1. AB5000 Ventricle commercially available for use as LVAD, RVAD, or , biventricular assist device.

wall to contain the pump chambers (Thoratec IVAD; Thoratec Corp, Pleasanton, CA, USA) or four blood cannulas (Berlin Heart Excor, Berlin Heart GmbH, Berlin, Germany; Thoratec BVAD, Thoratec Corp, Pleasanton, CA, USA; Abiocor, Abiomed Inc, Danvers, MA, USA) that penetrate the patient's skin. The latter carries an excessive risk for cannula or even mediastinal infection. Two implantable centrifugal LVADs from the HeartWare HVAD (HeartWareInc, Framingham, MA, USA) have also been used for biventricular assist.[23]

Percutaneous RVADs

The primary benefits of an implantable RVAD is optimal hemodynamic support that can be sustained over time. The disadvantages are those of any surgically implantable VAD, including the requisite operation and risks of infection, device thromboemboli, and bleeding. Given the capability of the RV to recover more rapidly and completely than the LV and the desire to avoid an operation, a minimally invasive percutaneous RVAD optimized for the treatment of potentially recoverable acute RHF is attractive.

A percutaneous RVAD should reduce the workload of the RV without the need for cardiotomy, minimizing trauma to the myocardium and affording the best possible chance for recovery. Due to the need for longer duration of support, percutaneous RVAD is not appropriate for destination LVAD therapy. However, for the acute heart failure group with potential for recovery, short-duration RV support may be adequate and desirable and, thus, could be attractive to allow the RV to recover in patients in whom LVADs are used for bridge-to-recovery and, possibly, even in those treated for bridge-to-transplantation. Percutaneous RVAD support would not be suitable for patients with chronic nonrecoverable heart failure who may need to wait several weeks to months until a donor heart is available for transplantation.

Percutaneous assist devices for RV failure

Although there is currently no percutaneous device specifically approved for right side in the United States, two novel devices have been used to offer percutaneous RVAD solutions.[22,24–27] They are (1) the commercially available TandemHeart percutaneous VAD (PVAD) device (Cardiac Assist Inc, Pittsburgh, PA, USA), which is approved for general circulatory support up to 6 hours; and (2) the Impella RP RV support system (Abiomed, Danvers, MA, USA), which is presently in clinical testing. These RV support devices differ in implantation technique, mechanism of action, maximal flow rate, and, thus, magnitude of hemodynamic support. They also differ in ease of insertion and potential complications.[24]

The TandemHeart PVAD was primarily designed for short-term mechanical LV support. The Tandem Heart involves the placement of a 21 F inserted into the left atria from the femoral vein via a transseptal puncture. Blood is withdrawn from the left atrium by an external centrifugal pump and infused into the femoral artery via a 14 to 19 F (**Figs. 2** and **3**). The Tandem Heart can provide up to 4.5 L/min of cardiac support. Because of the large catheter diameter, iliac-femoral angiography must be performed before cannula insertion.

Compared with the IABP, the Tandem Heart has been shown to improve hemodynamic parameters in two small trials.[26] However, there is a higher rate of complications with device use, including bleeding, tamponade, and vascular complications. The complexity of its insertion (>30 minutes in some cases) and higher complication rate compared with Impella or IABP has limited the use the Tandem-Heart in high-risk percutaneous coronary intervention (PCI) patients. Placement of the TandemHeart System does not require surgery, and can be done in the cardiac catheterization laboratory.

The TandemHeart has been demonstrated as a percutaneous assist device for RV failure in two cases.[3,4] The method involved placing two 21 F cannulae—one in the right atrium and another in the pulmonary artery (**Fig. 4**). Both femoral veins were used. A 7-F Berman wedge catheter from the right femoral vein was put into the right pulmonary artery and, then, using a long, extra-stiff guidewire, exchanging this catheter for the 21 F dilator and cannula. The skin and tissue tract were dilated before insertion of the 21 F cannula into the right pulmonary artery. A similar technique was used from the left femoral vein to insert a second TandemHeart 21 F cannula into the right atrium. The system was primed and an air-free connection was made to the pump circuit. At 3 L/min pumping,

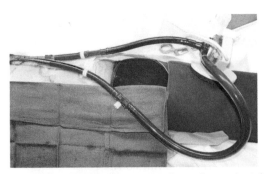

Fig. 2. The TandemHeart cannula and centripetal pump during hemodynamic support. The blue-tagged cannula draws blood from the left atrium to the pump, which returns it to the femoral artery cannula.

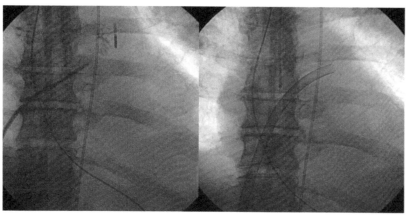

Fig. 3. Insertion of the tandem heart requires transseptal puncture (*left*) and dilation of the atrial septum followed by passage of the large cannula to the left atrium (*right*).

there was marked hemodynamic improvement with weaning of vasopressors and increased urine output. RV function assessed with serial ECG demonstrated gradual improvement.

However, because adequate left atrial pressures are required for sufficient pumping, the Tandem-Heart is contraindicated with any of the following: (1) predominant right ventricular failure, (2) ventricular septal defect, (3) aortic insufficiency, and (4) severe peripheral vascular disease. Currently there are no large studies and scant case reports

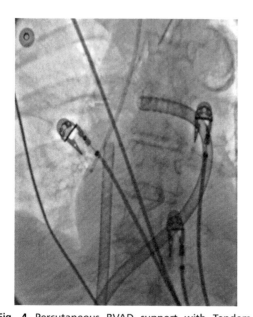

Fig. 4. Percutaneous RVAD support with Tandem-Heart device. (*From* Atiemo AD, Conte JV, Heldman AW. Resuscitation and recovery from acute right ventricular failure using a percutaneous right ventricular assist device. Catheter Cardiovasc Interv 2006;66:78–82; with permission.)

on use of the TandemHeart for RV failure in the absence of cardiogenic shock due to LV compromise.

Impella Percutaneous RV Support Device

Abiomed's Impella LV support platform has been adapted for primary use as a direct RVAD support device: The dedicated Impella RP RV support system design is based on the LV Impella 5.0 (Abiomed Inc, Danvers, MA, USA). In contrast to the TandemHeart centrifugal flow pump, the Impella LV support system uses a miniaturized axial flow pump fitted onto a pigtail catheter to directly unload the LV (as opposed to the left atrium) and delivers blood to the ascending aorta, simulating normal physiology.[24] These devices are the world's smallest LVADs and can be implanted intravascularly by interventional cardiologists in the catheterization laboratory and by surgeons in the operating room. The smaller (12F) 2.5 device can provide 2.5 L/min flow, while the larger (22F) 5.0 can provide 5 L/min flow at physiologic afterloads. The blood pump is powered by a miniature electric motor that is protected from blood flow ingress by a dextrose purge solution. Impella support for the LV differs hemodynamically from the TandemHeart[27,28] in that it directly aspirates blood from the LV and ejects in an antegrade fashion in the ascending aorta, thus avoiding the afterload increase inherent with the femoral retrograde outflow of the TandemHeart device. It is also technically easier to implant. Early studies suggest that the use of Impella 2.5 in support of high-risk PCI cases results in favorable short-term and mid-term angiographic, procedural, and clinical outcomes,[29] including in patients undergoing emergency PCI for ST elevation IMI.[30]

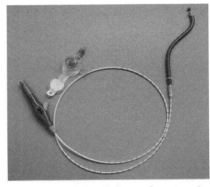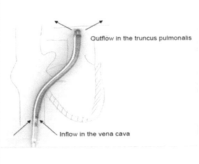

Outflow in the truncus pulmonalis

Inflow in the vena cava

Fig. 5. Impella RP pump catheter (*left panel*); anatomic placement of Impella RP (*right panel*).

Dedicated impella RV device

The Impella RP system is also a catheter-based design (**Fig. 5**) comprised of a 22F pumphead (electric motor, axial blood pump, and outflow cannula) mounted on an 11 F (see **Fig. 5**). It is capable of delivering flows up to 4.8 L/min for up to 2 weeks of support. The Impella RP is placed percutaneously through the femoral vein via the Seldinger technique using a vessel dilator, sheath introducer, and guidewire. The pump crosses the tricuspid and pulmonic valves in an antegrade fashion, with its inlet in the inferior vena cava and its outlet in the pulmonary artery just proximal to the bifurcation (**Fig. 6**). The entire procedure can be accomplished in approximately 10 minutes.

The Impella RP may offer clinical advantage based on its small size and surface area compared with commercially available extracorporeal RVAD systems. Compared with the currently available extracorporeal RVAD systems, Abiomed's AB5000 Ventricle (a pulsatile pneumatic blood pump) and the LevitronixCentriMag RVAS (Levitronix LLC, Waltham, MA, USA) (a centrifugal maglev blood pump), the Impella RP's blood contacting surface area is lower, the pump offers excellent surface washing characteristics due to its simple flow geometry and a novel speed modulation scheme.

The Impella RP system has been tested in chronic animal studies designed to assess biocompatibility and device function. Over a 14-day period of implantation, all devices functioned well and all animals survived to necropsy. There was no hemolysis, valve damage, pulmonary embolization, device thrombosis, infection, or organ dysfunction, and the devices were free of thrombus at explant.

First-in-man clinical feasibility evaluation has been initiated (in Canada and Europe) in patients experiencing RV failure in different clinical settings, including post-heart transplant, post-cardiac surgery and RV failure post-LVAD. To date, device implant was successful in all cases and the devices were extremely stable after initial positioning. The Impella RP delivers maximum flow of up to 4.8 L/min, though an average flow of 3.6 to 3.8 L/min was deemed adequate to support the patients. On initiation of support, the patients experienced improvement in clinical status and hemodynamics with a decrease in central venous pressure and increase in mean aortic pressure. RVAD support ranged from 1 to 7 days, with greater than 60% of patients supported for more than 4 days and explanted on RV recovery.

SUMMARY

RV failure is an increasingly common clinical problem that may require mechanical support. In contrast to severe LV failure, RV failure is

Fig. 6. Percutaneous RVAD support with Impella RP pump catheter antegrade across tricuspid and pulmonic valve, with inlet in inferior vena cava and outlet in pulmonary artery.

typically more reversible, therefore application of shorter-term percutaneous support devices is potentially attractive. Current innovations promise greater availability of such percutaneous RV support devices.

REFERENCES

1. Goldstein JA. State of the art review: pathophysiology and management of right heart ischemia. J Am Coll Cardiol 2002;40:841–53.

2. Bowers TR, O'Neill WW, Grines C, et al. Effect of reperfusion on biventricular function and survival after right ventricular infarction. N Engl J Med 1998;338:933–40.

3. Atiemo AD, Conte JV, Heldman AW. Resuscitation and recovery from acute right ventricular failure using a percutaneous right ventricular assist device. Catheter Cardiovasc Interv 2006;66:78–82.

4. Giesler GM, Gomez JS, Letsou G, et al. Initial report of percutaneous right ventricular assist for right ventricular shock secondary to right ventricular infarction. Catheter Cardiovasc Interv 2006;68:263–6.

5. Meyer P, Gerasimos FS, Ahmed MI, et al. Effects of right ventricular ejection fraction on outcomes in chronic systolic heart failure. Circulation 2010;121:252–8.

6. Banerjee D, Haddad F, Zamanian RT, et al. Right ventricular failure: a novel era of targeted therapy. Curr Heart Fail Rep 2010;7:202–11.

7. Fukamachi K, McCarthy PM, Smedira NG, et al. Preoperative risk factors for right ventricular failure after implantable left ventricular assist device insertion. Ann Thorac Surg 1999;68:2181–4.

8. Taylor DO, Edwards LB, Aurora P, et al. Registry of the International Society for Heart and Lung Transplantation: twenty-fifth official adult heart transplant report—2008. J Heart Lung Transplant 2008;27(9):943–56.

9. Lee S, Kamdar F, Madlon-Kay R, et al. Effects of the HeartMate II continuous-flow left ventricular assist device on right ventricular function. Heart Lung Transplant 2010;29:209–315.

10. Matthews JC, Koelling TM, Pagani FD, et al. The right ventricular failure risk score a pre-operative tool for assessing the risk of right ventricular failure in left ventricular assist device candidates. J Am Coll Cardiol 2008;51(22):2163–72.

11. Jett GK, Picone AL, Clark RE. Circulatory support for right ventricular dysfunction. J Thorac Cardiovasc Surg 1987;94(1):95–103.

12. Higgins RS, Elefteriades JA. Right ventricular assist devices and the surgical treatment of right ventricular failure. Cardiol Clin 1992;10(1):185–92.

13. Reiss N, El-Banayosy A, Mirow N, et al. Implantation of the Biomedicus centrifugal pump in post-transplant right heart failure. J Cardiovasc Surg 2000;41:691–4.

14. Moazami N, Pasque MK, Moon MR, et al. Mechanical support for isolated right ventricular failure in patients after cardiotomy. J Heart Lung Transplant 2004;23(12):1371–5.

15. Osaki S, Edwards NM, Johnson MR, et al. A novel use of the implantable ventricular assist device for isolated right heart failure. Interact Cardiovasc Thorac Surg 2008;7:651–3.

16. Law MA, Grifka RG, Mullins CE, et al. Atrial septostomy improves survival in select patients with pulmonary hypertension. Am Heart J 2007;153:779–84.

17. Rose EA, Gelijns AC, Moskowitz AJ, et al. Long-term use of a left ventricular assist device for end-stage heart failure. N Engl J Med 2001;345:1435–43.

18. Kormos RL, Teuteberg JJ, Pagani FD, et al. Right ventricular failure in patients with the HeartMate II continuous-flow left ventricular assist device: incidence, risk factors, and effect on outcomes. J Thorac Cardiovasc Surg 2010;139(5):1316–24.

19. Miller LW, Pagani FD, Russell SD, et al. Use of a continuous-flow device in patients awaiting heart transplantation. N Engl J Med 2007;357:9.

20. Hsu PL, Parker J, Egger C, et al. Mechanical circulatory support for right heart failure, 2011 mechanical circulatory support for right heart failure: current technology and future outlook. Artif Organs 2011. DOI:10.1111/j.1525-1594.2011.01366.x.

21. Shuhaiber JH, Jenkins D, Berman M, et al. The Papworth experience with the LevitronixCentriMag ventricular assist device. J Heart Lung Transplant 2008;27:158–64.

22. Anderson M, Smedira N, Samuels L, et al. Use of the AB5000 ventricular assist device in cardiogenic shock after acute myocardial infarction. Ann Thorac Surg 2010;90(3):706–12.

23. Krabatsch T, Potapov E, Stepanenko A, et al. Biventricular circulatory support with two miniaturized implantable assist devices. Circulation 2011;124(Suppl 1):S179–86.

24. Naidu SS. Novel percutaneous cardiac assist devices the science of and indications for hemodynamic support. Circulation 2011;123:533–43.

25. Vranckx P, Meliga E, De Jaegere PP, et al. The Tandem Heart, percutaneous transseptal left ventricular assist device: a safeguard in high-risk percutaneous coronary interventions: the six-year Rotterdam experience. EuroIntervention 2008;4:331–7.

26. Thomas JL, Al-Ameri H, Economides C, et al. Use of a percutaneous left ventricular assist device for high-risk cardiac interventions and cardiogenic shock. J Invasive Cardiol 2010;22:360–4.

27. Schwartz BG, Ludeman DJ, Mayeda GS, et al. High-risk percutaneous coronary intervention with the TandemHeart and Impella devices: a single-center experience. J Invasive Cardiol 2011;23:417–24.

28. Kovacic JC, Nguyen HT, Karajgikar R, et al. The impella recover 2.5 and TandemHeart ventricular assist devices are safe and associated with equivalent

clinical outcomes in patients undergoing high-risk percutaneous coronary intervention. Catheter Cardiovasc Interv 2011. DOI: 10.1002/ccd.22929. [Epub ahead of print].

29. Maini B, Naidu SS, Mulukutla S, et al. Real-world use of the impella 2.5 circulatory support system in complex high-risk percutaneous coronary intervention: the Uspella registry. Catheter Cardiovasc Interv 2011. DOI: 10.1002/ccd.23403. [Epub ahead of print].

30. Engström AE, Sjauw KD, Baan J, et al. Long-term safety and sustained left ventricular recovery: long-term results of percutaneous left ventricular support with Impella LP2.5 in ST-elevation myocardial infarction. EuroIntervention 2011;6:860–5.

Index

Note: Page numbers of article titles are in **boldface** type.

Moving?

Make sure your subscription moves with you!

To notify us of your new address, find your **Clinics Account Number** (located on your mailing label above your name), and contact customer service at:

Email: journalscustomerservice-usa@elsevier.com

800-654-2452 (subscribers in the U.S. & Canada)
314-447-8871 (subscribers outside of the U.S. & Canada)

Fax number: 314-447-8029

Elsevier Health Sciences Division
Subscription Customer Service
3251 Riverport Lane
Maryland Heights, MO 63043

*To ensure uninterrupted delivery of your subscription, please notify us at least 4 weeks in advance of move.

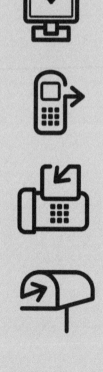

Printed and bound by CPI Group (UK) Ltd, Croydon, CR0 4YY

03/10/2024

01040351-0011